ART THERAPY WITH OLDER ADULTS

ART THERAPY WITH OLDER ADULTS

A Sourcebook

Edited by

REBECCA C. PERRY MAGNIANT, MA, ATR-BC

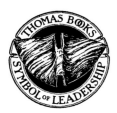

CHARLES C THOMAS • PUBLISHER, LTD.
Springfield • Illinois • U.S.A.

Published and Distributed Throughout the World by

CHARLES C THOMAS • PUBLISHER, LTD.
2600 South First Street
Springfield, Illinois 62704

©2004 by CHARLES C THOMAS • PUBLISHER, LTD.

ISBN 0-398-07456-9 (hard)
ISBN 0-398-07457-7 (paper)

Library of Congress Catalog Card Number: 2003061802

With THOMAS BOOKS *careful attention is given to all details of man-
ufacturing and design. It is the Publisher's desire to present books that are satisfactory as to their physical qualities and artistic possibilities and appropriate for their particular use.* THOMAS BOOKS *will be true to those laws
of quality that assure a good name and good will.*

Printed in the United States of America
CR-R-3

Library of Congress Cataloging-in-Publication Data

Magniant, Rebecca C. Perry
Art therapy with older adults
    p. cm.
ISBN 0-398-07456-9 -- ISBN 0-398-07457-7 (pbk.)
1. Art therapy for the aged.

RC 953.8.A76A78 2003
615.8'5156'0846--dc22

2003061802

CONTRIBUTORS

AMY BAKER, MA

MA in Counseling Psychology/Art Therapy from Naropa University
Boulder, Colorado

JOAN BLOOMGARDEN, PhD, ATR-BC, CGP

Director of the Hofstra University Graduate Creative Arts Therapy Program
Hempstead, LI, NY

PAMELA J. BRETT-MACLEAN, MA

Doctoral Candidate, Individual Interdisciplinary Studies Graduate Program,
University of British Columbia, Vancouver, British Columbia Canada
Researcher, Department of Family Medicine, University of Alberta, Edmarton,
Alberta Canada

LEE DORIC-HENRY, M.ED., ATR

Doctoral Student, Adler School of Professional Psychology, Chicago, IL

JAN FENTON, ATR-BC, LPC

Art Therapist / Psychotherapist at Renfrea of Southern CT, Wilton, CT, Center
for Hope, Darien, CT, and Private Practitioner in New Canaan, CT

LINDA LEE GOLDMAN, M.ED., ATR-BC

Adjunct Faculty, National Louis University, Wheeling and Evanston, IL
Private Practitioner and Art Therapy Consultant in Northbrook and Chicago, IL

MARILYN M. MAGID, BFA

Manager, Therapeutic Programs and Volunteer Services
George Derby Centre, Burnaby, British Columbia, Canada

REBECCA C. PERRY MAGNIANT, MA, ATR-BC

MA in Art Therapy from The George Washington University, Washington, DC
Former Director of Art Therapy, Goodwin House West, Falls Church, VA
Paris, France

EILEEN P. MCGANN, MA, ATR-BC

Senior Art Therapist, The Jewish Board of Family and Children's Services,
New York, New York
Faculty Adjunct, Graduate Art Therapy Program, New York University, NY, NY
Faculty Adjunct, Graduate Art Therapy Program, School of Visual Arts, NY, NY
Faculty Member, Art Department, Molloy College, Rockville Centre, NY

KATHLEEN MESSMAN, ATR-BC, RN, MPS

Naropa University, Adjunct Faculty
Colorado Department of Public Health and Environment, Health Professional II

SHINYA SEZAKI, MA

MA in Creative Arts Therapy, Hofstra University, Hempstead, NY
Akimoto Hospital, psychiatric unit, Chiba, Japan

JUDITH WALD, MS, ATR-BC

Art Therapist, New York Presbyterian Hospital, White Plains, NY
Adjunct Assistant Professor, College of New Rochelle, New Rochelle, NY

DENIS WHALEN, MA, OTR

Registered Occupational Therapist, Dominican College, Orangeburg, NY
Masters in Expressive Arts Therapy, European Graduate School,
Saas Fe, Switzerland
Director of the Living Arts Project of Glass Lake Studio, Albany, NY
Core faculty, Glass Lake Studio Expressive Arts Training Program
Adjunct faculty, Russell Sage College Occupational Therapy Dept, Troy, NY

INTRODUCTION

When I began my career working with older adults in art therapy (as an intern in my first practicum placement), my eyes were opened to the rich and varied experiences alive within a retirement facility. I learned that art can give insight, if only for a minute, into the mind of a person suffering from Alzheimer's. I learned that art can soothe anxiety and bring relief from depression. But most importantly were the life lessons I learned from the elders around me. I learned from their personal histories as if I were in the midst of a live history lesson. I learned that death, no matter how natural it may seam when someone is in their 90s, is always difficult to deal with. But I also learned to have hope. Hope that by bringing art therapy to a wheelchair-bound individual, I might brighten their minutes, their hours, their days, helping them to resolve whatever issues they may have. The issues ranged from the profound, meaning-of-life type, to the mundane, I-hate-the-food-in-this-place. But from each and every person, I learned a lesson.

The chapters in this book provide a wide range of information on working in art therapy with older adults. Our hope is that you will learn new ways of working with your clients, or better yet, be inspired to seek out a way to work with older adults if you do not already. Please also note the wide range of further resources listed in the Recommended Readings Section.

The Benefits of Art Therapy in your Facility

Art therapists are trained to provide clinical art therapy, but can also provide case management, assessment, development of treatment plans and goals, and staff inservices and education. Therapy can be particularly important for the older adult population, because as a person ages, the problems he/she has in life age along with him/her. Their issues are the same as the ones we have—from family and marital conflict, to abuse, depression, and anxiety. The difference seems to stem from the fact that older adults know that they have less time to face the issue. Thus, they look inwards, ". . . becoming less concerned with outer appearances and events and more absorbed in internal reflection," according to art therapist Susan Spaniol, in an editorial in the 1997 issue of *Art Therapy: Journal of the American Art Therapy Association*, vol. 14(3) They may finally have the time to look inside, perhaps at conflicts or emotions that they have held inside for decades. Art therapists, thus, can provide a nonthreatening means for self-expression and self-exploration through the art process.

Art therapists are masters-trained clinicians, and can be registered and certified by the Art Therapy Credentials Board (ATCB) after completing postgraduate supervised clinical hours and an exam. An art therapist can be hired contractually (from an hour a week to full time, ranging from $10-$100 an hour, depending on experience and setting), as part of a clinical team (along with social workers, psychologists, nurses, and psychiatrists), or as part of a therapeutic recreation department. The average salary for a full-time art therapist has a large range, due to the vastly different settings in which art therapists work. Although not a large proportion of art therapists work with older adults (only about 5% according to the American Art Therapy Association, Inc's 1998-1999 Membership Survey Report), the expectation is that the field, like many other health care fields, will continue to expand as the baby boomers move into long-term care. Art therapy can be a cost-effective method of relieving some of the plagues of nursing facilities, including depression, hopelessness, and grief. The discipline offers something new to those nursing facilities with other mental health practitioners, and can easily be incorporated into a program. We hope that this book inspires you to seek out art therapy for your facility, if you do not have such a program already in place.

R.C.P.M.

ACKNOWLEDGMENTS

First and foremost, I would like to thank all of the authors and practitioners who participated in this project. They all patiently stood by as I moved from one continent to another, with their chapters in hand. The process was truly a collaborative effort, and could not have been done without all of their insight and hard work.

I extend my sincere gratitude to my mentor in the field, Janet Beaujon Couch, for teaching me things about art therapy and life that cannot be learned in the classroom. To all of my other professors, colleagues, and clients, I thank you for the privilege of working with you.

Thanks also to my family for their constant support—my father for his experience in writing and publishing, my mother for her overseas research assistance, my sister for her editing advice.

Last, a huge *merci* to my husband, Stanislas, for keeping me on track and for being my biggest fan. This book would not be possible without you.

CONTENTS

ART THERAPY WITH OLDER ADULTS

SECTION I

ART THERAPY INTERVENTIONS AND IDEAS FOR WORKING WITH OLDER ADULTS

Chapter 1

POTTERY MAKING ON A WHEEL WITH OLDER ADULT NURSING HOME RESIDENTS[1]

LEE DORIC-HENRY

This chapter draws on research that I conducted in 1995 at a nursing home in Saline, Michigan.[2] The central focus of the study was to conduct qualitative and quantitative research to assess whether a sample of 20 older nursing home residents exhibited any changes in anxiety, depression, and self-esteem after an eight-week ceramics intervention using the Eastern method of throwing pottery on a potter's wheel. The main findings of this study were that the participating group showed significantly improved measures of self-esteem and reduced depression and anxiety, relative to a comparison group who did not participate in the art therapy intervention (Doric-Henry, 1995, 1997). In addition, those who showed the most improvement were the older adult residents with the lowest self-esteem and most depression and anxiety prior to the study. In this chapter, I explore some of the benefits and drawbacks of pottery making on a wheel with older adults. This chapter should: (a) help nursing home activity directors and fellow art therapists decide whether this is a worthwhile intervention for their particular populations; (b) provide a resource for planning based on the problems encountered in doing this type of art as therapy with older adults; and (c) provide insight into the problems and possibilities of making pottery with other populations, such as those with mental illness or physical handicaps, many of whose limitations are shared with older adults.

PREVIOUS RESEARCH

There is little published research on pottery-making on potters' wheels with older populations. In general, the literature contains two kinds of studies: (1) broad, but often unsupported statements expressing the value of art and creative crafts for older adults; and (2) empirical evidence from studies of art therapy interventions with older adults. The former are more plentiful than the latter.

The existing research on clay work with older adults focuses on hand-built pottery or crafts. These projects tend to use self-hardening clay or baker's dough rather than the "real stuff" which requires a kiln in order to be fired. This may be due to the lack of resources, a common complaint in most facilities. Literature about clay work with older adults includes instruction on pinch, coil, and slab work (Gould & Gould, 1971, Bodkin, Leibowitz & Eiener, 1976, Lowman 1992), but virtually nothing about working with clay on a potter's wheel. The majority of crafts suggested for use with older adults are simplistic, sometimes to the point of insulting the intelligence of the clients. This may be due to the author's experience with low functioning seniors, their need to do anything (meaningful or not!), and the result of society's lowered expectations and "infantalization" of seniors.

Although older adults in the community and in institutional settings suffer from many physical difficulties, these are often worsened by accompanying psychological problems such as low self-esteem, "anxiety, depression, somatization and conversion disorders, phobias, obsessive-compulsive, schizoid and passive-aggressive behavior" (O'Malley, 1988, p. 233). Further, O'Malley points out that disengagement theory indicates that in a society where the kind of activity undertaken is determined by age, society assigns older adults increasingly less responsibility. This contributes to a loss of status and self-esteem, with the result that noninvolvement leads to further deterioration, especially in depression and anxiety. Taylor (1987) has argued that art has a positive effect in counteracting the negative experience of ageism.

Literature on "art as therapy" suggests that a product-oriented approach is particularly appropriate when conducting art therapy with older adults (Miller, 1984). According to Gould and Gould (1971), older adults are highly motivated by being able to help others, especially children. They enjoy and get fulfillment out of being able to "do" for others. During my observations over the period of a year at the nursing home, it became clear that a significant motivation for creativity came from this "need to give" that is inherent in elders. As grandparents and parents they had previously been able to provide gifts to their offspring, relatives, and friends, and although gift giving is an established part of human social interaction (Mauss, 1954), because they are in nursing homes, older adults are often deprived of this important and meaningful activity.

The promise of ceramics products can fulfill the "need to give" as well as serving as an incentive to engage in a risky activity; one where failure looms, but success lures. It has been argued that "art-based activities of high quality often have a halo effect on social acceptance and self-esteem as they build skills" (Edelson, 1991, p. 82). Further, these activities are especially valuable for older adults. This has been recognized by their inclusion "as a staple of adult education courses and program activities in senior citizen facilities" (p. 83). Erikson, Erikson & Kivnick (1986) point out that art can be especially valuable to older adults because it provides sensory stimulation. Others have noted that producing high quality art is both possible and desirable for older individuals (Lewis, 1987).

As a physically challenging art activity, Gould and Gould (1971) have argued that creative crafts are especially valuable for older adults. But they say, "when we become older and our hands and eyes are weakened through age and illness, many of our old skills are lost" (p. 3). At this time in the life course, the motivation for creativity might be lost with the loved ones who inspired it. Gould and Gould (1971) suggest that time "becomes virtually an enemy once there is little purposeful activity to fill the hours" (p. 3). They conclude that a good craft program in a nursing home can provide "a socialization experience for the patients" and help them to "become part of a group by working with others". But importantly, also, a craft program can help residents with their physical difficulties: "Some crafts can serve a dual purpose by also offering physical therapy. . . . Crafts can be a 'fun way' to increase hand coordination and mental concentration" (Gould & Gould, 1971, p. 3). This appears to be especially true for pottery. When older adult participants in the pottery project began to focus on their artwork, they took on the personas of "potters at work," intent upon production, how many objects to make, who to give it to, what color it should be, what it would be used for. Their progress and intent in pottery was similar to that of their needlecraft sessions but more intense. For needlecraft they employed familiar techniques and materials. Now they were in a new world, one of surprise and wonder, not just with the media but also with themselves.

When the therapist first introduced them to their pottery sessions, she began with some history about pottery. She told them about the Southern United States potters whose families lived and gained their livelihood from digging their own clay and selling their wares. For many, pottery offers a new learning experience, a connection with the history of their culture, and an opportunity for growth and discovery through the use of clay as an art media. For older adults, these effects can be enhanced since involvement in the process of pottery demands full attention of the mind and body, and it employs the artist's senses entirely. "The innate-enhancing effect of art-based activities can enhance self-images under siege by the double stigmas of old age and disability" (Edelson, 1991, p. 81).

It is also important to distinguish between the client's ability and "learned helplessness" (Jefferson, 1987) that can affect many older individuals. Indeed, evidence on self-esteem and older adults suggests "self-esteem (or the lack of it) leads to a set of personal-social expectations that generates a self-fulfilling prophecy. The result is a decrease in creative contributions even when, from an abilities point of view, such creative contributions are still potential if unrealized" (Jaquish & Ripple, 1981, p. 117).

Some limited support exists concerning the value of clay projects with older adults. For example, King and colleagues (1987), used a slab method to build a pottery village, to which each resident added their own house as well as shops and a church. This proved a delight and inspiration for older adult stroke patients. Moreover, in their hand-building efforts, the subjects attempted to use their stroke-affected sides.

It has been argued that those with visual impairment, which afflicts older adults to varying degrees, can also benefit from pottery. Ceramics offers a tactile feast–the feel of the cool, wet, smooth clay spinning around at speed controlled by one's foot on the pedal. The wheel responds to every nuance much like a sewing machine or race car and its effect is felt by the body. Indeed, "Ceramics and weaving, due to their tactile nature, are both highly suitable to people who are legally blind. . . . Ceramics can readily be taught to individuals with visual deficits, who often have heightened tactile abilities. . . . Verbal directions and the use of physical models are particularly helpful in guiding the creation of the final product for individuals who are visually impaired" (Edelson, 1991, p. 88-89). Edelson further argues that, "For people with poor hand strength or poor motor coordination, ceramics can help build vital skills. Manipulation of the clay can build motor abilities. The malleability of clay allows individuals with poor motor skills to correct mistakes in construction without ruining products and experiencing the additional frustration of making irrevocable errors" (pp. 89-90). Participants in my own research study included two residents who were blind. Interestingly, I noted that both did more work with their hands, even on their thrown pieces, than the other participants.

How an art intervention, including pottery, is designed is very important to its success. It is necessary to build the activities one at a time. Edelson (1991) explains that in this way "each day provides guaranteed success as well as a stretch into new activities and skills. Repeating activities and allowing sufficient time for project completion are essential elements in the design of the program" (p. 90). She also states that "these methods provide opportunities for learning and success which will enhance poor self images and encourage individuals to attempt and master new tasks" (p. 91). Reflecting upon Edelson's writing, I am reminded of one particular resident who told me she felt like she was "in college" when she participated in the project. She explained that when she was younger she always wanted to go to college and taking this "class" made her feel like she had fulfilled a part of a long-dormant wish.

Given this general positive acclaim for the psychological and physical therapeutic effects of art and pottery with older adults, it is perhaps surprising that little empirical research is focused on evaluation of its effects. There is some positive evidence from controlled art therapy studies with institutionalized older adults that shows support for the notion that art intervention stimulates creativity (Wikstrom et al., 1994), improves one's level of "happiness, peacefulness, satisfaction and calmness" and reduces one's level of depression and sense of despair (Wikstrom et al., 1992, 1993). Art therapy with older adults is also claimed to help older people verbalize their feelings and past experiences and to reinforce their autonomy (Callanan, 1994). Evidence suggests that creative art activity with disabled older adults provides them the opportunity to make decisions which can improve their originality, individuality, independence, self-concept and self-image, while facilitating stress reduction and coping skills (Aspell, 1976; Foster, 1992). However, while art therapy with older adults has been widely discussed (Callanan, 1994; Dewdney, 1975; Harlan, 1990; Miller, 1984; & Rugh, 1985), "the body of literature on developing art programs for the institutionalized elderly is relatively small" (Weiss, Schafer & Berghorn, 1989, p. 10). Further, "with few exceptions. . .the literature has lacked systematic analysis of the impact of arts programming on elderly students" (p. 11).

An exemplary study of art therapy's impact on the institutionalized older adults in a nursing home is that conducted by Weiss, Schafer, & Berghorn (1989) in which an eight-week textile painting class was evaluated using a quasi-experimental design. This study demonstrated that the art therapy intervention significantly improved social interaction among the high functioning residents and that the quality of art work improved during the intervention. However, Weiss, Schafer, and Berghorn found no significant improvement in the participants' self-esteem, although they point out that this may be a result of their participants having high pre-test self-esteem and that they may have already reached a self-esteem ceiling. Overall, the authors conclude that arts programming in nursing homes contributes to the social well-being of the residents.

Unfortunately, very limited direct empirical evidence exists in the literature specifically concerning the value of doing pottery as art therapy with older adult residents. As Yaretzky, Levinson and Kimchi (1996, p. 76) observe, "there is scant reference to geriatric rehabilitation using clay as a therapeutic tool." These authors have provided one of the best studies to date. Their research was conducted on eight older adult patients hospitalized with stroke and femur neck fractures who were participants in a five-week pottery group intervention project designed to improve their physical and psychosocial rehabilitation. They argue that working with clay "enables sensorimotor therapy for the upper limbs and fosters visual-motor coordination, spatial perception and construction and communication" (p. 76). Based on retrospective observation of videotaped sessions and a qualitative questionnaire, they found that the intervention improved sensorimotor skills. It also proved stimulating, allowed tension relief through the expression of feelings, and promoted fellowship, cooperation, and support (Yaretzky, Levinson & Kimchi, 1996, p. 76). However, these researchers were unable to determine the precise therapeutic effect of working with clay relative to contributions from other dimensions of the group process; they call for more evaluative research (p. 81).

In the research reported here, an attempt is made to evaluate the dimensions of well-being for pottery making with institutionalized older adults. In this study, 20 older adult nursing home residents (average age 83.5) were found to reduce their anxiety and depression and improve their self-esteem after an eight-week ceramics intervention using the Eastern method of throwing pottery on a potter's wheel. The control group was a group of 20 residents (average age 85.9) who did not participate in the art therapy intervention (Doric-Henry, 1995, 1997). In addition, and partly explaining the "ceiling" effect found in Weiss, Schafer and Berghorn's 1989 study, those participants in the present study who showed the most improvement were older adults with the lowest self-esteem and most depression and anxiety prior to the study.

THE NURSING HOME SETTING

The Evangelical Home is a church-supported 240-bed facility. Most residents are older adults ranging in age from their 70s to 100s. Many residents reside in a state of reasonable comfort at the nursing home for as long as ten years or longer. Some are admitted as couples, man and wife, and share a room together; all efforts are made to make the residents feel at home. There is no limitation on visiting hours. Friends and family members, including children and pets, are a frequent sight.

Although the nursing home is Evangelical in its affiliation, people of all races, nationalities, religions and denominations are welcome. The population is divided into two distinctly different groups: able-bodied and wheelchair or bed-bound. Those who are able-bodied (not needing assistance with activities of daily living or with wheelchairs) are situated in separate independent living quarters. These residents are free to come and go from the building and to choose those activities that they would like to attend. Other residents are able to walk with the assistance of walkers or canes; however, a large portion of the residents are confined to wheelchairs or to bed. Many residents who are wheelchair-bound are not able to toilet or dress themselves without assistance, but are otherwise capable of many normal activities. Range of hand and arm movement in many is very good. They are encouraged to attend "volley balloon," cane, and aerobic groups which keep those moveable body parts in action rather than allowing the residents' bodies to atrophy. The busy activity calendar offers the residents many choices, something very important to older adults. This is supported by other studies (Foster, 1992).

The Resident Population

Residents at this facility were typically housewives and mothers who were not formerly employed outside the home. Many had lived on farms. Their interests included: gardening, cooking, sewing, needlework, and music, among other things. The physical health of the residents ranged from good to extremely poor. Residents suffered chiefly from: crippling arthritis, strokes, incontinence, cancer, and broken bones. Psychological diagnoses of residents included: mild depression, dementia, Alzheimer's, and organic brain damage, though many were institutionalized for solely medical or physical reasons such as high risk of falling.

Of those who volunteered for the research project and agreed to become participants in the pottery sessions, some were "regulars" at other activities such as the studio art, craft, and needlework groups. Their willingness to explore uncharted territory indicated that they had potential as successful potters. Although their handicaps would seem to most pottery instructors to be impossible obstacles, those interested were not excluded because of physical limitations or disabilities. As a result, residents with strokes, arthritic and shaking hands, blindness, etc., were included in the group. Some residents who ordinarily attended only a small number of activities, but who were expected to substantially benefit from pottery were also singled out and approached to join the group.

The unusual mix of participants was inspired by the philosophy of the Activity Department's then Director, Kim Phelps. She reasoned that the high functioning older adult residents had freedom of mobility and comfortable living quarters (one of these residents even did carpentry in his room and others drove their own cars). The terminally diagnosed residents (last stages of Alzheimer's, etc.) could have their quality of life improved for the time we spent with them, but otherwise may be physically incapable of even the simplest functions such as intelligible conversation or feeding themselves. These residents received regular scheduled one-to-one visits by therapists, activity staff, and Harvey, the hardest working rabbit in Saline, Michigan. The remaining large and diverse population who, in spite of Alzheimer's disease, dementia, crippling stroke effects, blindness, and physical handicaps, was able to benefit from art therapy. This group's quality of life can be vastly affected, and this was the group I chose to target in my project.

In summary, the population of older adult residents selected for the study was comprised of 20 participants (average age 83.5) with an age range of 50 to 95, 19 of whom were female, one male. The 20 non-participants were of an average age of 85.9, with an age range from 76 to 99 years, 16 of whom were female, and four male.

EASTERN METHOD THROWING AS AN ART THERAPY INTERVENTION

There is an important difference between "Western" and "Eastern" method throwing. Western method throwing is the pottery technique used by many art teachers in the United States. One lump of clay is centered, formed, sliced off the wheel, and is ready for drying, firing, and glazing. This method requires a great deal of practice in order to center a piece of clay. In order to use the Western method, it would be necessary to center a new piece of clay each time a participant was successful or unsuccessful. Thus, the therapist would probably spend more time preparing the clay than the subject spent working on it. Due to time constraints and physical limitations of the population, this method was ruled out as the therapist had personally experienced the pain and frustration it affords during her first pottery experience in undergraduate school.

The Eastern throwing method (Beittel, 1989) has several advantages over the Western method, which make it especially appropriate as a technique to use for older adults. First, and most important, it was easy for the residents to learn compared with the Western method because a large amount of clay has been precentered and preformed by the therapist and older adult potters are able to work on another piece after having made the first, without the therapist needing to throw and center more clay. This method allows the therapist to initially center a 4 1/2 lb. piece of clay which is used by the client, one "knob" at a time, allowing the client four or five opportunities for success before a new lump of clay must be centered.

The centered clay is then built into a tower shape. A small door-knob shape is formed at the top of the mound. The client is then instructed to insert their thumb into the center of the knob as far as it is comfortable. If they find this motion difficult, the index and middle finger can be used together to open the top. The thumb, which is now centered inside the knob, is then pushed outward, and raised up from inside of the pot, putting pressure on the inside while the other hand supports the structure from the outside. To bring up walls, pressure is applied on the inside and outside of the piece (see Figure 1-1). The clay must be kept constantly wet while working. A sponge or wet hands are used in order to build up a layer of slip on the outside of the piece while working on it; however, water cannot be allowed to accumulate in the bottom of the piece or it will become too soft, so a sponge is used to gently remove excessive water from the bottom. Both hands are necessary to shape the clay while squeezing it firmly and evenly.

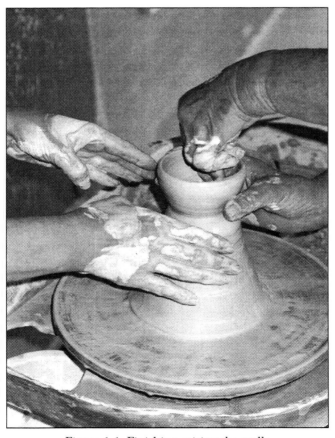

Figure 1-1. Finishing raising the walls.

Adapting the Eastern Method to the Nursing Home Setting

In the nursing home research, the therapist provided a "second hand" for stroke victims with use of only one hand. Too firm a pressure with both hands causes an excessively thin area that can result in the pot collapsing or tearing from the wheel. By keeping her hands on the opposite side of the pot, the therapist was able to feel most disasters and help the potters correct them before their pieces were ruined. The participants had never potted before, and therefore undertook the activity with great care. As a result, potential disasters were prevented because the speed at which the participants proceeded was much slower than speeds used by the ordinary potter.

Finished pieces were removed from the site, and taken to the therapist's home for drying, trimming, and bisque firing as the nursing home had no kiln (see Figure 1-2). The therapist carefully documented each piece, photographing each pot before and after trimming, during glazing and then the final product (see Figure 1-3). Glazing was done by the participants before the final firing. This is the stage where the potters had the most fun. We worked together as a group and each potter saw what their cohorts had been working on for the first time.

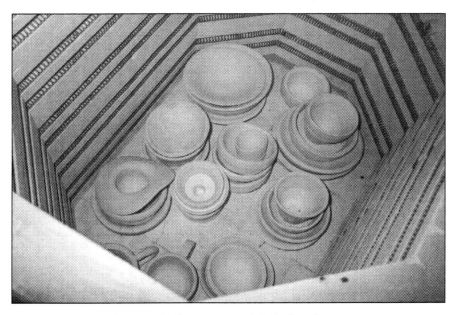

Figure 1-2. Greenware in kiln before firing.

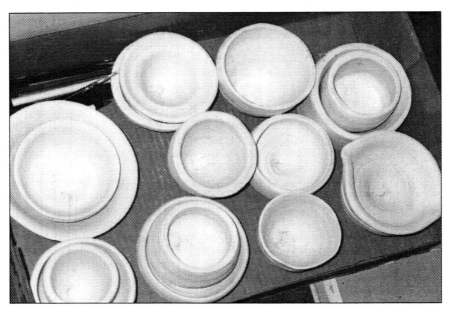

Figure 1-3. Unglazed bisqueware.

While potting, the participants gained confidence. They were encouraged to proceed with increasingly less instruction and intervention, and as their sessions progressed, some potters were able to complete an entire piece with very little assistance. Wherever and whenever possible, they were encouraged to work independently. In the beginning, the process of pottery-making was explained to the residents. Participants at first were invited to feel the clay as it spun within their cupped hands and to feel the slip build up on its surface. Next came placing an indentation, centrally located, on the top of the clay knob. The therapist guided their fingers to its center. If that failed, she made a small indention herself and guided their finger into it. Then a thumb or two fingers were pushed downward into the hole. Overall, clients appeared not to have difficulty doing this although they proceeded at a slow pace. The next step was to widen the hole and then to begin to raise the walls of the object. The clients were encouraged to experience the feel of the clay, and the focus was on this process rather than the pressure to produce a specific object.

The first experience one has with clay is usually memorable. There is no other media quite like it. The clay resists at first. When approached, it is a hard unruly wad, an insurmountable mountain. For the beginner, centering seems as impossible a task as climbing Mt. Everest. The therapist precentered a 4 1/2 pound block of clay, a difficult task for most beginning potters, thus allowing the Eastern method of throwing to afford older adults passage into a world inhabited by the much more experienced potter. With pressure and the synchronization of both hands, a shape begins to emerge and finally, the clay yields completely and blossoms into a beautiful shape.

Besides the wheel-throwing described above, two other uncertainties were similarly surmounted. First, low fire clay was chosen, which, due to its relatively low firing temperature requirements, averted accidents and catastrophes associated with high fire clay such as melt downs, cracking, and explosions. Also, white grogless clay was chosen rather than red to avoid regressive associations. The grogless clay was used in order to spare the delicate skin of the potters. (At one point, the therapist had to substitute a finely grogged clay and the potters not only noticed, but said it hurt their hands.) Secondly, a commercially available, low fire, predictable glaze was chosen. The therapist went a step further to ensure that the glaze colors chosen by the residents resulted in fired colors that were the same, by preparing small test tiles which she affixed to the top of the glaze jars, and having the clients choose colors from those rather than from a color chart. Having personally experienced all of the above mentioned frustrations which pottery can heap upon the novice potter, the therapist concluded that older adults would not have their lives enriched by similar experiences.

THE POTTERY INTERVENTION

The sessions consisted of individual one-on-one instruction in using a potter's wheel to form relatively small objects such as mugs, cups, and bowls. Care was taken to prepare the clay prior to the session in order to afford the maximum productivity, learning experience, and opportunity for success to the participant. The sessions designed as "art as therapy" were described to the clients as pottery classes. The eight sessions offered were approximately 50 minutes long, including wheeling or walking the resident to the session, pottery making, clean-up and returning the resident. The study was designed to include taking the potter through the entire ceramics process of wedging, throwing, drying, trimming, bisque firing, glazing, and glaze firing so that by the end of the classes they would have totally completed at least one piece and have experienced the hypothesized benefits of the art intervention. (See Figure 1-4.) Materials and equipment employed included: low fire white clay, bamboo knifes, steel kals, various shapes of wooden ribs, natural sea sponges, wire, potter's wheels and a kiln. Several plaster bats were prepared by wrapping the wheel head with a band of thin metal and lining this with plastic wrap. The supplementary plaster bats, which could be attached with clay to the steel wheel head, allowed the therapist to remove them from the potter's wheel with their pots intact, to use a new bat, and continue the session.

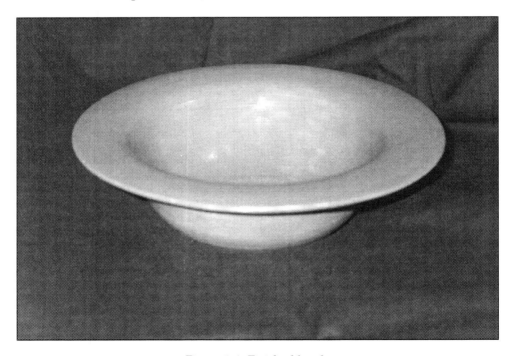

Figure 1-4. Finished bowl.

Most residents needed physical assistance to and from the activity room, which was provided by the therapist. It was not possible for the Activity Department to lend anything more than moral support and encouragement (which were offered in abundance) to this project as they were understaffed themselves. A crucial requirement for participation in this project was that the older adult potters had enough strength and mobility in their hands to execute forming the clay. Dr. Park, an advisor on the project, suggested opening the piece with two fingers instead of the thumb in order to reduce cramping of the hand. This worked well for several potters.

When experienced potters are about to lose a piece because it has gone out of control, become too large or wide, they will sometimes call another potter to their wheel and together "choke" the piece applying four hands to reform the errant clay. While working with the clients I occasionally employed Edith Kramer's (1986) "Third Hand" technique, actually beginning the piece or following the client's instructions when the residents were reluctant to participate; and furthermore, the potter's "fourth hand" was used to save wayward pots.

The setting for the pottery sessions was a large, well-lit, meeting room which doubled as part of the Activity Department. Placement of the potter's wheel was next to a large picture window looking out onto a grassy knoll. There was a large sink for washing up and participants had the company of Harvey (the nursing home's resident rabbit) and two parakeets. When this area was not available it was necessary to move the potter's wheel, tubs of water, towels and ceramic tools into a lounge in another part of the building.

Preparation for the project required that the potter's wheel be operational and that several plaster bats be readied for use as mentioned earlier. Petroleum jelly and plastic wrap were used between the bat and wheel head originally, but with little success. It appeared that a more substantial material such as metal might need to be used. In the end, reshaped pizza tins worked best since the metal conformed well to the shape of the wheel head but was easily removed after the plaster was set. Making six plaster bats allowed the therapist to precenter several pieces of clay each day, which could be set aside and used when clients needed them.

Indicative Case Studies

Space precludes discussion of the 20 case studies that were part of the original study. Below I have selected three case studies which are indicative of both the themes and the problems of conducting an art therapy pottery intervention with this client group. The names of the clients are fictitious. The full accounts of these cases are contained in Doric-Henry (1995). Three conventional assessment instruments were administered (Beck Depression, Coopersmith Self-Esteem, State-Trait Anxiety) to the participants. The effect of the intervention for each of the clients is discussed below at the end of each case with the complete results for the results for all the clients relative to the control group reported in Doric-Henry (1997).

Case 1: "Lucy"

Lucy was an 88-year-old wheelchair-bound former nurse who had previously suffered from depression, but showed no evidence of this at the time of the study. Lucy was very lucid and understood the directions; however, her nails were too long and she wanted them cut. Her hand strength and coordination were good, and she had a positive attitude, followed instruction well and showed no aversion to clay.

Lucy came to the second session without a reminder or encouragement from the therapist. She started right in without instruction and opened the clay well. She had difficulty getting her hands in the correct position to raise the walls of her piece, even with prompting and demonstration. Lucy had difficulty understanding which fingers went inside the pot and which to place outside. She was lucid and talked about previously suffering from depression, saying that her son had recently taken her to a psychiatrist. She explained that she attended too many activities "and pottery too" to be depressed. She complained that the antidepressant made her sleepy, and that she was not currently depressed. She showed no aversion to clay and insisted on cleaning up very well before leaving.

Before another session, when picking up Lucy from her room, the therapist was asked to read a story she had written. (This was the third occasion that Lucy had asked the therapist to read it.) She recalled incidents from her nurse's training during our trip to the activity room, saying that our (the nursing home's) nurses did a good job. When we arrived at the Activity Room and began potting, she was able to open her piece without directions. She produced a short medium-size symmetrical bowl and was especially pleased with its graceful shape. She remarked that it would be a surprise to her sister to find that she had been doing pottery, as Lucy's only aptitudes previously were cooking and work. She commented that now that she was in the nursing home she had time to attend gardening, exercise, music, etc., comparing these to all the clubs her sister belonged to. It seemed that the pottery was giving a boost to her self-esteem.

At the next session, Lucy stated that she would rather come to pottery than to Bingo (to the amazement of the therapist!). Again, as in previous sessions, she began well with little instruction and worked independently, but still appeared to have difficulty with placing her thumbs outside and other fingers inside the clay. She pressed with her thumb and appeared not able to relax it. The therapist put her hand outside the piece and under the client's thumbs. Lucy continued to follow instruction and produced a symmetrical, medium sized bowl. She was able to finish the piece with verbal instruction and approximately ten percent intervention by the therapist while recalling past memories of box lunches during eighth grade. She began to reminisce, and several references were made to her life on the farm as a youngster and to nurse's training later in life. She appeared relaxed, in a good mood and showed no aversion to working with clay or waiting with slip-laden hands for water to clean up. Lucy showed independence in clean-up, doing 50 percent of the work herself. She remarked, "This is fun. I wish I had learned to do this a long time ago."

At this session, Lucy decided to make a lid for the bowl made at her previous session. Given several options, she decided to make a domed lid. She had no difficulty understanding the concept of hollowing out the lid once it was sliced from the mound and placed atop her bowl. She watched the therapist demonstrate with a clay tool and was able to use the tool herself without assistance. Lucy discussed concerns she had about her roommate who had had a stroke and was unable to use one hand, saying that she had encouraged her roommate to begin sewing again. The therapist agreed this was a good idea. Lucy continued with her pottery, was pleased with the fit of the lid and chose to make a ball- shaped handle for it.

Today, Lucy chose two pieces to glaze and decided to make the outside and inside of each one different colors. She applied the glaze carefully and very slowly, talking throughout the session. She had to be listened to very carefully as she had misplaced her bottom dentures. Themes of food, raising children, and her sister were recurring but with new details. Lucy expressed a wish to help her roommate and the therapist explained she could bring a special plaster project the next day, which Lucy could help her roommate to paint as an Easter project for her roommate's grandchildren. The qualitative expressions indicating a positive experience with the art therapy intervention were supported somewhat by the objective data. Lucy's score on the Coopersmith Self-Esteem Inventory slightly improved from 80 at pretest to 84 at post-test and her scores on State Anxiety Inventory declined from 24 to 20. Interestingly, there was no change on the Beck Depression Inventory scores, which were 0 at both pre- and post-test, indicating no depression.

Case 2: "Mildred"

Mildred was an 85-year-old former employee of a psychiatric hospital. Mildred showed great potential for this intervention; her hand strength and reflexes were excellent. She was good at following instructions, unsure of herself at first, but willing to try. She was easy to work with, pleasant, and happy. After the first session she joked, quite pleased with herself, "I guess I'm not ready to die yet. I just learned something new!" The client also stated that she enjoyed the feel of the clay and did not mind the mess. She talked about her former job at a Ypsilanti mental institution and how much she enjoyed it. She made a mug without a handle and said she preferred it like that to drink her coffee. Lily, a nursing home friend, who watched quietly throughout the session, accompanied her.

In today's session, Mildred cheerfully agreed to come for her session accompanied again by Lily. She dug right in and did a great deal of the work herself. She was very pleased with the shape of her pot. Therapist demonstrated the necessary movement that the client was able to imitate well, but without much pressure.

Today, Mildred did 80 percent of the work herself. She opened the clay about an inch too deep but was able to follow other instructions. She was not able to remember what she made last time (neither could the therapist) and asked if she could make something for her granddaughter who was very interested in all the things she did. "This is fun. I like this. I like to keep busy. I go to all the activities. I'm learning something new every day!" Her affect was bright and she was in a jovial mood. She was able to raise the clay walls without too much difficulty and was curious about when the pots would be "done" (to give to people).

In this session Mildred brought another resident with her who was severely affected by Alzheimer's. Mildred appeared very distracted today. She opened the clay well but went too deep into the center of the piece, nearly to the wheel head. When attempting to raise the walls, she became confused and dug a finger into the outside of the pot. The therapist was about to repair the accident when it occurred to her that Mildred had just created a terrific candleholder. When Mildred studied it she not only agreed, but also liked the piece. We decided to "quit while we were ahead." Mildred cleaned the piece with a sponge following instructions not to put pressure on the piece but to allow the sponge to drag across the surface to mop up excess debris and slip. The Assistant Activity Director entered the room and expressed great approval, both surprised and amazed at Mildred's accomplishment. Mildred could not decide right then what color the finished piece should be glazed but said she'd think about it.

At the next session Mildred was again accompanied by Lily, who was quiet and observed without interruption throughout the session. Mildred accomplished approximately 60 percent of the work herself. She remembered how to begin and followed instruction well. Mildred decided to make a bowl and was assisted by the therapist to widen the opening and raise the walls. The client followed verbal cues to finish the piece with a sponge. Mildred was pleased with the finished piece saying, "I didn't know I could do anything like that!"

In today's session Mildred applied glaze carefully pulling out stray brush hairs. She told a story about a former psychiatric patient (for the fifth time). She was able to remember names, locations, and occupations of grandchildren. Mildred said she planned to give the piece she was glazing to her granddaughter "because she likes handmade things." Again, qualitative expressions of a positive experience with the art therapy intervention were supported somewhat by the objective data. Mildred's score on the Coopersmith Self-Esteem Inventory improved from 88 at pre-test to 96 at post-test and her scores on State Anxiety Inventory declined from 24 to 20. No change was recorded on the Beck Depression Inventory scores, which were 0 at both pre- and post-test, indicating no depression.

Case 3: "Gloria"

Gloria was an 87-year-old blind resident of the nursing home who was physically frail and prone to falls. Gloria did not feel well physically but was in a very good mood. She agreed to try the potter's wheel in her room "to get an idea" of potting. She felt the wheel, wheel head and clay and kept feeling the clay as it was formed into a shape while showing no aversion to the slip. She also felt the hole in the center and tried with her finger to deepen it without being asked. She worked at the bottom of the piece after it was thinned out and kept working on its sides. After the wheel stopped, she squeezed the clay for another five minutes. She did not like the shape (organic and fungus-like), so she kept working on it. She exclaimed, "The clay feels icky but I like it." Gloria was very happy and talkative. She asked the therapist to describe the shape (this time like a calla lily). Gloria said that she wanted to come to the Activity Room next time, instead of working in her room. She also was worried about water splashing off the wheel, and other difficulties with the space.

Gloria arrived early for today's session in the activity room. Though blind, she asked for instructions and found her way down the hallways to the Activity Room by herself. She had several obstacles and some people in wheelchairs to circumvent on the way, but she appeared pleased with her independence. She potted in the darkened room where a movie was being shown and asked several times about what pictures were being shown, which residents were attending, and what each was doing. She was eager to begin and able to follow instructions. She said, "I don't want to make a piece of junk." When her piece had its walls raised, she began to work with them while they were stationary, producing a piece similar to her first one. Gloria worked with the clay for quite a while but was unsatisfied. Finally, the piece became too soft and the therapist explained that it would need to sit for a couple of hours in the open air to firm up and would be brought to her room to finish. When this was done, the client said she did not like the piece as much as her first.

Gloria had requested a particular color glaze for today's session and the therapist located some in the apple green color she had asked for. Gloria did her glazing with a small, fine-textured elephant-ear sponge which was provided instead of a brush so that she might be able to feel the piece as she was glazing it. The therapist steadied the glaze jar and Gloria was able to find it each time without much difficulty. She covered 85 percent of the surface without assistance. She joked about being a potter and how the pot would look on her son's desk when it was finished. Gloria asked the therapist whether potting was something blind people could "do." The therapist replied that working with clay was recommended as an art activity for the blind because of its tactile nature and explained further that many times the therapist looked away or closed her eyes when working on her own pottery in order to get a true feel of the piece and to reassure herself that it was centered.

On the next occasion, the therapist brought Gloria's pot to her. She said she liked how it felt. She had fallen over the weekend and had broken two ribs and a bit of spirit as well. She winced with pain when she tried to move and was distressed about the fall, concerned about the ensuing operation and worried that her son and daughter-in-law were moving. Gloria improved on all three measures, pre- to post-test: Coopersmith 68 to 76; Beck 3 to 1; State 40 to 36.

MEANING OF POTTERY MAKING TO OLDER ADULTS

In addition to the objective measures, the researcher also constructed a short subjective questionnaire with some open-ended questions. Based on the open-ended qualitative survey given to the 20 older adult participants, I was able to get a good sense of what this intervention meant to them. Most found the overall experience to be "fun," "exciting," and a "joy," especially compared to the routine of their daily lives. As one resident said, "It gave me something to do. I was sitting here looking at the walls and it kind of depressed me. . .it helped me. I was surprised that I could create anything like that." Indeed, for many, the satisfaction of the pottery intervention came from meeting the challenge of gaining new knowledge and achieving new accomplishments. "It was exciting for me because I'd never done it before," said one of the participants, while another said, "It was something I thought I couldn't do, creating something like that and I loved it." For another, the fact that she was involved in pottery was pleasantly surprising. "It was like amazing that I should be doing something so different. . . . I was proud that I could handle such work, especially learning to do it for the first time in my life. I enjoyed every minute and it was really interesting." Others said "I think I achieved something," and "I feel great. I got a love for pottery from doing it," and, "I made something I thought I couldn't make. It gave me a good feeling." One resident said, "I was proud that I had the courage to get into it." Another reflected that "I can do pottery now. I was the one who had most things done."

Yet it was not simply the overall accomplishment that enriched these older adult lives, but also the physical, kinesthetic interaction with the medium. One resident described feeling "like a little kid playing in the mud. I wanted to eat it." Another expressed satisfaction that it allowed her to "use my hands" following a stroke. Yet another observed that "Working with your hands helps a lot and some people sit all day almost in a catatonic state." Yet some, especially initially, "didn't like how it felt." At first, the feel of clay was different and uncomfortable: "soft and cold" and it got "underneath my fingernails (and) felt uncomfortable," "like dirt in my hands," said one resident. However, once they became familiar with this sensation, residents adjusted. "Even though I got my hands dirty, it washed off." As another said, "I had to get used to it. I didn't like it at first because it felt so gooey."

Several of the residents commented that working with clay had a much broader benefit than its immediate intrinsic rewards. One pointed out that the activity focused the mind on something positive, whereas another recommended pottery making to other nursing home residents, saying that it "would make them more confident," make them "feel better." As yet another said, because "those people who can't do anything would have the incentive that they're creating something and it would make them feel better." One resident said, "It made me feel that I can go on to bigger things."

Not missing the entrepreneurial opportunities pottery-making offers, a few saw the economic potential in making clay pots for sale. However, it was the pleasure in others' reactions to their pottery making that provided an additional reward, partly from being able to surprise their family with such an accomplishment, and partly by making something of creative value enabling the act of giving. "My daughter got a bowl and she thought it was great. She loved it." "My friends and my son thought it was great." "They were really happy I made stuff like that and were interested in it." Another resident responded, "They thought it was great when I made that vase. My granddaughters said

'Oh grandma you made wonderful things.'" "I told my children and they were really happy that after all these years (as a retired person) I was learning something."

One 95-year-old resident decided her ceramic creation should be an Easter basket. She asked the therapist to bring Easter grass and candy. Together we arranged the basket, which she hid, with mischievous elfin-like glee, in her dresser drawer. She surprised her daughter with it on Easter Sunday. The therapist later discovered that the resident hadn't told her daughter she was participating in the project, so it must have been quite a surprise!

The overall statistical data (Doric-Henry, 1997) was supported by the qualitative statements made by the participants, and confirms that what the existing research suggests is true about art therapy, is also true for pottery as art therapy.

The Outcome of the Pottery Intervention

The statistical results of the quasi-experimental art therapy intervention have been reported elsewhere (Doric-Henry, 1997). In summary, the findings were that, relative to the comparison group, the pottery intervention significantly reduced depression for the older adult participants, significantly improved participants' self-esteem, and made a significant reduction in anxiety (state and trait). In addition, the therapist was interested to see whether these results were consistent with the findings of Weiss, Schafer & Berghorn (1989), who had found no significant improvement in self-esteem through their art intervention. However, they argued that because of the significantly higher self-esteem of the participants it was possible that the lack of significant improvement "reflects a ceiling effect." They state, "There may not have been much room for improvement in the self-esteem of participating individuals whose self-esteem, relative to their peers, was already high prior to participation" (Weiss, Schafer & Berghorn, 1989, p. 15). Weiss, Schafer & Berghorn's participants not only had high self-esteem prior to the intervention, but were physically capable as well. In contrast, this project, which included residents with a wide range of both physical and mental disabilities, allowed a broader spectrum of older adult subjects for analysis. Indeed, those with initial high self-esteem showed no significant improvement in self-esteem as a result of the pottery intervention. In contrast, those having a relatively low pre-test self-esteem showed a significant improvement. This result supports the findings of Weiss, Schafer & Berghorn (1989), and suggests that those with low self-esteem are likely to benefit most from art therapy interventions. The same procedure was also applied to the measures of depression and anxiety, with similar results (Doric-Henry, 1995, 1997).

Based on the qualitative data, the overwhelming majority of the participants found that making pottery was both a valuable and enjoyable experience. By answering the specific questions on the pottery evaluation, they lent credence to the therapist's original hypothesis that older people could make pottery if they used the Eastern method of throwing, and that it would improve their sense of well-being. During the course of the intervention, the therapist observed that the potters were becoming more independent and showing a sense of accomplishment in their work. Most of the potters were able to get used to the feel of the clay after a few sessions and even recommended the activity to others. Relatives and friends voiced their support. The Activity Department staff, as well as volunteers, all reported that they had heard the residents talking about how much they enjoyed doing pottery. Even Helen, a long-time janitorial staff member, said "I'm so happy to see them (the residents) doing things like this!"

Contrary to the therapist's preliminary fears about raising the potters' anxiety, the use of the Eastern method accompanied by physical assistance enabled most of the potters' perception of their anxiety to not increase. The majority of potters also reported that after making pottery they felt good about themselves and that they felt happy. Making pottery, perhaps because it is not age-defined, presented an opportunity for the Saline potters to be something other than "old."

CONCLUSION AND DISCUSSION

One of the most important discoveries of this particular project was the necessity to not pre-judge the client's ability. A number of the potters included in the study would have been eliminated if physical ability had been the criteria. With lots of patience and assistance these potters were able to create and grow. On the whole, this group made the largest strides in improvement of ability. Those potters who were very capable from the start did well throughout the sessions and tended to outproduce the others in both quality and quantity. However, from the standpoint of sheer enjoyment and satisfaction, the two subgroups of potters did not appear to differ. Wheelchairs were a problem, but the majority of wheelchair-bound potters were also able to sit in ordinary chairs safely. Due to the often small size and weight of older adult participants, it was possible for the therapist to transfer them without mishap. Once seated, they were able to pot in the same position as a real potter, and to obtain similar results! The white low-fire clay was ideal for most of the participants. However, for one client even this was too regressive. If red clay had been used, she probably would not have made it past the first session. For one potter with severe arthritis and swelling of the hand joints, the motion of the wet clay against the skin of her hands produced a prickly sensation which felt like a million tiny "needles." The participant was very apologetic that she could not continue, but the therapist responded that her experience was extremely valuable in a "scientific" sense, in that it provided information that was important about older adults with arthritic hands. She smiled and said she was worried that her hands might be a problem but was pleased that she had at least tried.

For the most part, the potters became more and more independent as the sessions progressed. By the end they were arriving at sessions ready to pot with sleeves rolled up and jewelry removed. A transfer routine from wheelchair to regular chair became familiar and expected. Constant hand-cleaning that had been evident in several potters during their first sessions abated by the fourth or fifth session. Potters also evolved from sitting at the wheel passively waiting to be toweled off after the sessions, to taking an active role in clean-up. The more mobile potters stood up, walked to the water bins and washed their gooey hands without instruction. Even negative reactions to the slip and ongoing jokes about the "messy" business of potting, also subsided by about the fourth or fifth session.

However, depth perception emerged as a common problem. Unable to properly judge by sight where to stop, the potters were pushing further downward than the bottom of the "knob" they were working with, making it necessary to carve away the underlying clay in order to accommodate the potters' bottoms. Doing this necessitated a great waste of clay and slowed down the potting process. Dr. Park, the project's ceramics consultant, recommended filling in the bottom of their pots with additional clay, and he gave the therapist instructions to make a small wooden tamping tool which would make it possible to fill the holes while pushing air bubbles out of the bottom.

Unfortunately, the potters' success in throwing did not carry through for all of them when it came time to glaze their creations. Poor eyesight that did not interfere with potting became a frustration some of them when attempting to glaze. For many it was a struggle to even get the paintbrush into the jar of glaze, let alone onto the pot. Poor eyesight was a trial, but some residents were legally blind and one, totally blind. Through trial and error with the blind participant, the glazing problem was overcome with a small sea sponge and mop brush which enabled the potter to feel the piece while glazing.

Motivating older adults to take part in a pottery program took enormous persistence. Two participants who repeatedly declined most of their sessions finally became interested during the eighth week of the study. The health of participants was also a major factor to consider. Frequently some of the residents were ill for extended periods of time, or were hospitalized. The entire institution was in quarantine for a short period due to an influenza epidemic, which brought the project to a halt for a short time.

Though the research conducted for this study yielded some promising data and implications, further work is necessary in order to validate the expenditure of energy and funds for a pottery program versus, for instance, a less costly form of art therapy that may yield similar results. Two important factors affecting the success of future research of this nature are the cooperation and commitment of the activity and/or supervisory staff and the availability of adequate accommodation for the ceramics sessions and equipment. The selected nursing home had the former, but lacked the latter.

It appeared that some participants derived more benefit from the pottery intervention than others. A crucial matter to investigate is the profile of those older adults that would benefit most from this intervention. Although this study was quite small, it did suggest that nursing home residents who are willing to participate report a sense of enjoyment and accomplishment from making pottery. Observation by the therapist and staff at the nursing home, as well as the outcome of the quantitative data analysis, supports this finding. It is the hope of this researcher that subsequent studies could be designed to answer this question.

Other recommendations for future study include having more research assistants. Though sample size in this study was minimal for statistical relevance, it was overwhelming for one therapist/researcher. Future studies of even this size require the assistance of an additional therapist or research assistants, because of the strenuous, labor-intensive demands of the pottery intervention and the physical assistance required by this population.

If a similar study is to be undertaken, it must also be noted that the issues of transference and countertransference cannot be ignored. Due to the nature of instructing older adults, which necessitates verbal and nonverbal interaction as well as physical contact, it would be crucial to constantly remind the client that they are participating in a time-limited project. Likewise, it is important to recognize that the sudden withdrawal of the therapist may have negative effects on the client. I continued as a volunteer worker at the nursing home and was fortunate to meet a local potter, who became interested in my pottery project and offered to volunteer at the site and to join the therapist in potting with the residents on a bimonthly basis.

Although the research and analysis was limited in scope, my overall impression was that this project was a distinctly positive experience for the participant potters, and an enlightening if exhaustive experience for the therapist. As indicated, this conclusion was supported both by the qualitative and quantitative data which showed that the participating group of older adults showed significantly improved self-esteem as well as reduced depression and anxiety, relative to a comparison group (Doric-Henry, 1995, 1997). In addition, those who improved the most were the older adult residents with the lowest self-esteem and most depression and anxiety prior to the study. The results suggest that nursing home activity directors and art therapists could introduce a program of pottery with older adults, provided that there are sufficient human and material resources available. In the case of limited resources, volunteer potters could be recruited and given thorough training by the art therapist in working with older adults. Moreover, it is recommended that further research using pottery making as an art therapy intervention be done, perhaps incorporating quasi-experimental design to evaluate its effectiveness. The research could also be implemented with other populations, such as those with mental illness or physical handicaps, many of whose limitations are shared with older adults.

NOTES

1. Several people have been very supportive in giving me advice in conducting this project. In particular I thank: Dr. Holly Feen, Dr. Arthur Park, Dr. Richard Sinacolla, Dr. Shlomo Sawilowsky, Dr. Talib Kafije, all from Wayne State University; Dr. Monroe Friedman from Eastern Michigan University; Dr. Robert Enright from the University of Wisconsin-Madison; and Dr. Dora Dobrin from Virginia Wesleyan College. I would also especially like to thank Kim Phelps, formerly of the Evangelical Home of Saline, and the late Marti Hoestra, its Activity Director during the time I was there, for their support and encouragement. Finally, I thank the elderly potters of Saline.

2. Pre- and post-interviews were conducted with each of the 20 participant and 20 nonparticipant comparison group residents. Pretests were conducted in February before the beginning of the pottery intervention. Pottery sessions were held February through April, 1995 and posttests were conducted in April. The tests consisted of standard preprinted questionnaires. The adult form of the Coopersmith Self-Esteem Inventory (Coopersmith, 1981) is comprised of 25 questions presented in true-false style, which evaluates self-attitudes. The Beck Depression Inventory (Beck et al., 1961) contains 20 questions measuring behavioral indications of depression. The State-Trait Anxiety Inventory (Spielberger et al., 1983) is composed of two 20-question sections designed to distinguish between general and present anxiety. Although some of the tests were designed to be self-administered, they were developed for populations with much better hearing and eyesight than the sample being used. As a result, the therapist administered the tests in one-on-one sessions, usually in the resident's room. Confidentiality was assured and the tests results were recorded using assigned sequential numbers, rather than names. In addition, qualitative methods were also employed. Evaluation notes were based on observations made while the participants took part in the pottery sessions. These notes were descriptive of behavior, artistic progress, problems, comments, and recommendations for further sessions. These notes were written following the sessions on the same day and were organized by participant number and chronologically ordered. In this way, the accumulated accounts show the progress of the participating potter, which culminates in their own self-evaluation of the sessions based on the qualitative questionnaire. At various stages of the intervention, photographs of the process were taken which depict the equipment, the setting, the set-up, various stages of the potters work, and some glazed pottery. Additional general data on the clients was obtained from the nursing home's charted information on residents and was summarized above. It was decided that given

the easily identifiable and sensitive nature of the residents' conditions, and in the interests of preserving client anonymity, specific charted data on individual clients would not be presented.

REFERENCES

Aspell, A. (1976). Why art education for the elderly blind? *Educational Gerontology, 1*, 373-78.

Beck, A. T., Ward, C. H., Mendelson, M., Mock, J., & Erbaugh, J. (1961). An inventory for measuring self-esteem. *Archives of General Psychiatry, 4*, 561-71.

Beittel, R. (1989). *Zen and the art of pottery*. New York: Weatherhill.

Bodkin, C., Leibowitz, H., & Eiener, D. (1976). *Crafts for your leisure years*. Boston: Houghton Mifflin Company.

Callanan, B. O. (1994). Art therapy with the frail elderly. *Journal of Long Term Home Health Care: The PRIDE Institute, 13(2)*, 20-23.

Coopersmith, S. (1981). *Self-esteem inventories*. Palo Alto, CA: Consulting Psychologists Press.

Dewdney, I. (1975). An art therapy program for geriatric patients. In E. Ulman, & P. Dachinger, (Ed.), *Art therapy in theory and practice* (pp. 126-131). New York: Schocken Books.

Doric-Henry, L. (1995). *Art as therapy: Eastern method ceramics as a therapeutic intervention for elderly nursing home residents*. Unpublished master's thesis, Art Therapy Program, Wayne State University, Michigan.

Doric-Henry, L. (1997). Pottery as therapy with elderly nursing home residents. *Art Therapy: The Journal of the American Art Therapy Association, 14(3)*, 163-171.

Edelson, R. (1991). Art and crafts - not "arts and crafts": Alternative vocational day activities for adults who are older and mentally retarded. *Activities, Adaption and Aging, 15(1-2)*, 81-97.

Erikson, E., Erikson, J., & Kivnick, H. (1986). *Vital involvement in old age*. New York: W.W. Norton.

Foster, M. T. (1992). Experiencing a "creative high." *Journal of Creative Behavior, 26(1)*, 29-39.

Gould, E. & Gould, L. (1971). *Crafts for the elderly*. Springfield, IL: Charles C Thomas.

Harlan, J. E. (1990). The use of art therapy for older adults with developmental disabilities. *Activities, Adaption and Aging, 15*(1-2), 67-79.

Jaquish, G. A., & Ripple, R. E. (1981). Cognitive creative abilities and self-esteem across the adult life-span. *Human Development, 24*(2), 110-119.

Jefferson, M. F. (1987). Essential adult educational programs in the visual arts. *Art Education, 40*(4), 32-41.

King, P., Shering, J., Kingstone, E., & Ingram, I. (1987). Using pottery with elderly people. *British Journal of Occupational Therapy, 50*(11), 384.

Kramer, E. K. (1986). The art therapist's third hand: Reflections on art, art therapy and society at large. *American Journal of Art Therapy, 24*(24), 71-86.

Lewis, H. P. (1987). Art and older adults: An overview. *Art Education, 5*, 41.

Lowman, E. (1992). *Arts and crafts for the elderly: A resource book for activity directors in health care facilities*. New York: Springer Publishing Company.

Mauss, M. (1954). *The gift*. London: Cohen and West.

Miller, B. (1984). Art therapy with the elderly and the terminally ill. In T. Dalley (Ed.) *Art as therapy: An introduction to the use of art as a therapeutic technique* (pp. 127-139). London: Routledge.

O'Malley, W. T. (1988). *Art therapy sourcebook.* Flint, MI: William T. O'Malley.

Rugh, M. M. (1985). Art therapy with the institutionalized older adult. *Activities, Adaption and Aging, 6*(3), 105-120.

Spielberger, C. D., Gorsuch, R. L., Lushene, R., Vagg, P. R., & Jacobs, G. A. (1983). *State-Trait Anxiety Inventory (form Y): Self-evaluation questionnaire.* Palo Alto, CA: Consulting Psychologists Press.

Taylor, C. (1987). Art and the needs of the older adult. *Art Education, 40*(4), 8-15.

Weiss, W., Schafer, D. E., & Berghorn, F. J. (1989). Art for institutionalized elderly. *Art Therapy, 6*(1), 10-17.

Wikstrom, B., Theorell, T., & Sandstrom, S. (1992). Psychophysiological effects of stimulation with pictures of works of art in old age. *International Journal of Psychosomatics, 39*(1-4), 68-75.

Wikstrom, B., Theorell, T., & Sandstrom, S. (1993). Medical health and emotional effects of art stimulation in old age: A controlled intervention study concerning the effects of visual stimulation provided in the form of pictures. *Psychotherapy & Psychosomatics, 60*(3-4), 195-206.

Wikstrom, B., Ekvall, G., & Sandstrom, S. (1994). Stimulating the creativity of elderly institutionalized women through works of art. *Creativity Research Journal, 7*(2), 171-182.

Yaretsky, A., Levinson, M., & Kimchi, O. L. (1996). Clay as a therapeutic tool in group processing with the elderly. *American Journal of Art Therapy, 34*, 75-82.

Chapter 2

THE USE OF SANDTRAY WITH OLDER ADULT CLIENTS

AMY BAKER

As part of a master's program in art therapy at Naropa University, I completed a 700-hour internship at a senior residence that provides independent and assisted affordable housing. A central part of the work revolved around using the sandtray as a therapeutic tool with individuals and groups. I found it to be highly effective in working with older adult clients in this setting. Here, I will attempt to provide a brief theoretical and practical background on the sandtray as a psychotherapeutic modality, focusing on the use of sandtray with individuals, including two case examples.

SANDTRAY BACKGROUND

Traditional Jungian Sandplay Therapy

Weinrib (1983) describes the use of the sandtray in traditional Jungian sandplay therapy: the client is not given a directive, and the therapist encourages the client simply to follow his/her heart, or to experiment (p. 12). A landscape or scene might emerge, a story might be enacted, or the client may simply play with the sand. The freedom allows the client to bring forth any aspect of his/her inner world that might need to be expressed.

After completing the sandtray, the client speaks about what he/she sees. The therapist might ask the client questions about the tray, or request that the client tell its story. The client may talk about memories triggered by the process. He or she may decide to make changes in the sandtray after talking about it.

At this point, the therapist usually has ideas about what the figures might represent in the client's psyche, but does not share these ideas until several sessions and sandtrays have been completed. He/she looks at the tray as a reflection of the client's inner mental and emotional state, and notes the archetypal figures that appear. The therapist has in mind a framework of the developmental stages of sandtray therapy, and carefully observes the client's behavior and creations with this framework in mind, but does not, at this point, share this information with the client. Only when the client has been immersed in the creative process over time, and experienced the healing which often comes from the process alone, does the therapist bring the "expert opinion" into the work (Weinrib, 1983).

The archetypes and their associated meanings and stories are resources for the therapist and later will become resources for the client. When the time is right, the therapist will share information about the figures, especially those that have appeared repeatedly in the client's sandtrays.

Directed Sandplay Therapy

Tennessen and Strand (1998) describe the differences between traditional sandplay therapy and directed sandplay, which has recently come into use, particularly with trauma survivors. In directed sandtray work, the therapist often asks the client to work with the figures in specific ways, such as holding one and asking it questions which are suggested by the therapist. The therapist might also ask the client to describe the sandtray with a certain approach in mind, such as a cognitive approach, which would focus on factual description without emotional content. Hence, with directed sandplay, the therapist orchestrates the process. He/she assesses the capacity of the client to move into different stages of a structured approach, first making sure that resources are strongly in place before touching on any traumatic material. This framework is based on the belief that healing is possible in a short-term, highly structured therapy context, while traditional sandplay is aimed at a lengthier process guided by the free rein of the client's psyche.

Sandtray as a Contemplative Practice

Working with the sandtray can be a wonderfully soothing and calming experience. Simply touching the sand brings one into a quieter state of mind. Weinrib (1983) calls it a form of meditation, and says that it has a centering effect similar to working with mandalas (p. 69). The physical containment of the wooden box promotes focused attention and "a state of absorption and relaxed concentration" (p. 69). Mindfulness is a natural byproduct of engagement in this process.

The habitual patterns of thought quiet down, and images, impulses, and narratives emerge from the unconscious as a sense of playful spontaneity takes over. The sandtray experience cultivates awareness of parts of the self that normally do not have a voice. Despite its apparent simplicity, the sandtray provides a glimpse into the workings of the unconscious. It invites the participant to drop into a nonordinary state of consciousness in which deep material may surface.

SANDTRAY WORK WITH OLDER ADULT CLIENTS

Getting Started

The traditional minimum requirement for a therapist to use sandtray with clients, according to Caprio (1993), is that the therapist has done a series of his or her own sandtrays. One can also go much further than this, getting supervision from an experienced sandtray therapist with training in teaching the Jungian sandtray approach.

The sandtray is a wooden box, 28 1/2 by 19 1/2 inches, three inches deep, filled halfway with sand. The inside of the sandtray is painted a medium shade of blue, and waterproofed if possible. Make sure to use sand that is safe for indoor use (available at home and garden stores). Many therapists have two trays, one for dry and one for wet sandplay. I used a single tray, and found it convenient to keep the tray on a cart, which could be easily moved from room to room, with a collection of figures stored on lower shelves. The figures range from about one-half inch to four inches tall and include: animals (farm, wild, birds, fish, mythological); people (babies to older people, multicultural); fantasy figures (mythological, popular culture, fairy tales); buildings (houses, churches, stores, schools); modes of transportation (cars, planes, boats, bicycles, trains); and objects from nature (shells, stones, feathers, sticks). Yard sales, toy stores, hobby shops, and Internet sites geared specifically to sandtray and therapeutic toys are great resources for starting a sandtray figure collection, which is truly a lifetime process. A collection might eventually include several hundred figures.

Ideas for Approaching Sandtray with Older Adult Clients

The therapist might tailor the way the sandtray is presented to the individual client. One resident loved collecting miniatures, and I introduced the sandtray initially as a way of sharing interest in a mutual hobby. Another was a writer, and the sandtray became a tool for getting started on a story.

Some older clients might see it as demeaning or infantilizing to be asked to "play with toys in a sandbox." It is important for the therapist to frame the experience as more than, and different from childhood play.

Ways to Work with the Sandtray

- the client writes a poem, short story, fairy tale, or descriptive paragraph about the completed sandtray
- the client creates a dialogue between two sandtray figures
- the client tells the therapist what he/she sees in the sandtray, what memories it brings up
- the client gives a title to the sandtray
- the client points out which object is most important in the sandtray
- a family member comes into a session and does a sandtray with the client
- a group of older clients create a sandtray together based on a theme such as loss or community

Goals of Sandtray Work with Older Adults

The goals of art therapy with the geriatric population often differ from those used with other age groups, due to the incredible amount of loss this group has experienced (Schexnaydre, 1993). Offering a modality with a high probability of success and satisfaction is one way to offset such losses in some small way and to provide opportunities to feel capable, confident, and proud.

Schexnaydre (1993) sees the goals of art therapy with older adults as improving quality of life and building on strengths. The soothing and enjoyable qualities of sandtray address the first of these. One can do sandtrays specifically about strengths, asking the client to choose objects that represent resources in his or her life.

Life Review

According to Schexnaydre (1993), life review is a way for older adults who have experienced loss after loss to remember and think about times when they felt capable, happy, empowered, and loved. There may be little or no interest in rehashing the past or resolving old issues; on the other hand, reliving happy memories and past successes can be quite beneficial. The sandtray is a nonthreatening medium through which older adults can create scenes from childhood or any life stage.

Addressing Developmental Work

The sandtray provides an individual with a forum to work with developmental issues of aging and facing mortality, whether at a conscious or unconscious level. Erikson (1986) characterizes the last stage of human development as an internal tension between integrity and despair. He describes integrity as "enduring comprehensiveness . . . a lifelong sense of trustworthy wholeness" (p. 55). Despair is "dread and hopelessness . . . bleak fragmentation" (p. 55). He does not say that the successful outcome of this tension is integrity, but rather a balance between the two, a synthesis of the opposites. The sandtray, like art-making in general, provides the opportunity to find symbols that represent opposites, and then find ways for them to coexist. Erikson describes the strength of this stage as wisdom, "detached concern with life itself, in the face of death itself" (p. 37). Sandtray allows one distance from an issue, a new perspective. Erikson also discusses the concept of "generativity" (Chinen, 1985, p. 52), in which there is a shift in values from one's individual concerns to interest in helping the community and future generations. I have seen this theme surface spontaneously in the sandtrays of older clients.

An openness to seeing the complexity in each situation is an aspect of Erikson's model of elder wisdom, as is flexibility and strength in the face of inevitable loss. The sandtray provides a forum to identify and explore strengths and work with multiple aspects of an issue. Erikson describes the central challenge as the ability to remain actively engaged, both in close relationships and the in world in broader terms. Work done in the sandtray session can ripple out into other aspects of the individual's life, opening the door for new ways to engage in living.

Case Example 1: Katherine

At the time of our work together, Katherine was 81 years old. Her husband had died 18 years earlier from Alzheimer's disease, which had been affecting him significantly since his early fifties. Katherine had one daughter who lived near her and with whom she had a very close relationship. She had had two other babies who were premature and died a few days after birth. Katherine had become a prolific writer in her later years.

I asked Katherine to create a sandtray and to write a fairy tale based on the tray. The structure of a fairy tale, with its conflict and resolution, seemed to be an ideal format for the issues that surface in this stage of life, as discussed above. By bringing the sandtray into fairy tale form, we allow safety through distancing the material in the realm of story. Themes which would be difficult or impossible to discuss directly can be addressed and pondered, and a resolution within the imaginal world could at some level aid in the real world struggle of an individual (Bettelheim, 1977). Katherine's sandtray (Figure 2-1) contains a group of figures arranged in a circle next to a bridge, around a small, red box with a key on top of it. The figures, listed clockwise, are: a dragon, a crab, a fish, a rooster, a rabbit, a man, a woman, and an older woman. All the figures face inward toward the box and key, with the exception of the fish, which faces the rooster to its left. The figures are clustered in the center of the tray, with empty sand surrounding them.

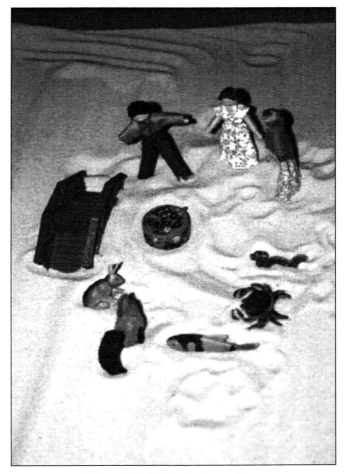

Figure 2-1. Katherine's sandtray.

After completing the sandtray, Katherine wrote the following:

Once upon a time there was a man and his wife who lived in a small village in China. This couple had been married for several years but had not had the child they longed for.

One day they decided to walk to a neighboring village where there lived an old woman who was known for her ability to predict happenings. When they reached the village the old woman took them into her cottage. She asked many questions about why they wanted a child of their own. When she decided to help them she gave them a red box with a key to open it. She also told them they could open the box only after they had done a good deed. But the couple did not pay heed to her direction.

Over the next few months they opened the box many times, but they found only strange creatures: a rooster one time, a rabbit another, a crab, a fish, a dragon.

The couple grew angry with the old woman. If she was able to make all these creatures come out of the box, why couldn't she make a baby come out? But this couple forgot all about the good deed they were supposed to do, and they never found out that was why they couldn't have a child of their own.

The sandtray made by Katherine had a ritual quality to it, a gathering of forces around a central element; as a whole it forms a mandala. There is an empty box at the center of the circle and an empty expanse of sand surrounding the small gathering: emptiness inside and out. This imagery reflects the theme in the story of the childless couple. A key rests on the empty box, and the old woman in the story tells the couple that the key to having a child is doing a good deed. In their haste to realize their dream, however, they forget this essential piece of information, symbolically losing the key to happiness.

Rather than a baby, the box produces a series of creatures. Katherine said, "The animals are still there—maybe they stay to haunt the couple." Failed attempts at fulfillment remain like ghosts; regret and loss are tangible in this world.

On an individual level, Katherine seemed to be using the sandtray and writing to revisit and to attempt to gain a sense of closure about an issue in her life. This reflects Katherine's process of life review, a developmental task of aging discussed by Schexnaydre (1993). The tale takes place in China, allowing Katherine to distance the story from herself doubly: first in the imaginal realm, and second geographically. Biographical details confirm her personal experience with having lost babies, and the story seems to express a belief or fear that she had done something wrong or failed to do something good, which resulted in these losses.

Katherine appeared to be choosing to face harsh reality rather than end the story with what she might see as a traditional "escapist" fairy tale ending. Was she expressing the despair Erikson describes? Another view would be that in her representation of this unresolved personal issue, she was doing the work of this developmental stage, attempting to come to terms in her own way with life's inevitable losses.

The tray and story do not offer guidance in resolving these feelings, as there is no resolution in the traditional fairy tale sense. The ending reflects no change or growth in the characters. Perhaps Katherine expresses the view here that there is no fairy tale ending; realistic acceptance of life's harshness replaces tidy closure. Katherine's meticulous style did not prepare me for this. I see it as a strength that she was able to tolerate the lack of resolution.

On a collective level, the story depicts a world that has forgotten the wisdom of the elder. Katherine, an elder herself, may be expressing what she sees as a societal theme. If she is the elder in the tale, her words fall on deaf ears, and the gifts she offers go to waste. A sense of powerlessness pervades the story.

Symbol amplification of Katherine's sandtray figures reveals parallels between her story themes and her choice of objects. The box can be seen as "a female symbol of the unconscious and the maternal" (Chevalier, 1996, p. 116). On one level, it is a perfect choice for a surrogate womb; at the same time, the barrenness can be seen as belonging to the psyche.

Both the rabbit and the fish are symbols of fertility and rebirth. The rabbit is an ambivalent symbol; it is lucky and unlucky, fertile and barren, and represents both plenty and wastefulness. The rabbit's familiarity with the unknown and unattainable makes it a go-between for humans to the "transcendent realities of the other world" (Chevalier, 1996, p. 472). Not only has the couple lost a child; they have missed the opportunity to touch the realm of spirituality.

Katherine, most likely, was unaware of the layers of meaning contained in the figures she had chosen. As therapist, I remained an observer at this stage. If a particular figure were to appear repeatedly over a series of sandtrays, I would tell her a bit about the mythology connected with it. For now, however, the primary focus was between the tray and its maker.

In the next session, Katherine spoke about her upcoming eye surgery, how she had not been sleeping well, and how anxious she had been feeling. I told her that another way of using the sandtray was to place objects in it that represent feelings or worries, as a way to put them outside oneself and get some distance, perhaps some new perspective. I asked her whether she would like to try this. She agreed. This second sandtray (Figure 2-2) contains a young woman who stands among keys, shells, a horse, a feather, a watch, and palm trees.

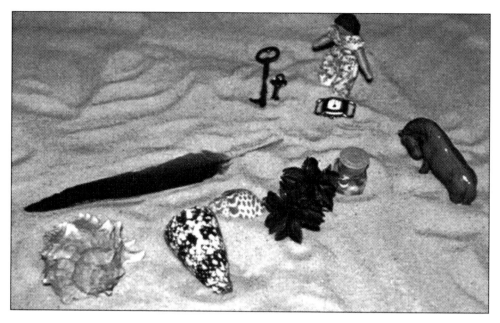

Figure 2-2. Another sandtray by Katherine.

Katherine wrote

This is [Katherine]. She's sad and worried because she doesn't have much time left. She's 81. The keys next to her are doors that are already closed for her. She knows that one easy way would be to just ride off into the sunset. Not suicide or anything like that, but to close her mind. Stop being really alive. So riding off on the horse isn't the option [Katherine] wants. . . . She wants instead to keep learning, opening to new things. To spend time doing what she loves, like bird watching. This is exciting to her not just because the birds are so beautiful, but because they are part of the whole cycle of things. And to walk on the beach, where she feels so peaceful.

She knows she has the urge or temptation to put things in these neat, square bottles like always. Fear, regret . . . but that's not how she wants to use the time left to her. So she's stopped worrying about whether–not whether, but *when*–she's going to die.

Katherine expressed difficult feelings here without trying to change them or bottle them up. Instead she acknowledged that they can exist alongside positive things. Her ability to look at loss simultaneously with good aspects of life reflects the developmental work she was doing, balancing integrity and despair as described by Erikson.

In processing the impact this work has had on me, I have been painting response pieces to each participant. The five animals that spontaneously appeared in the painting (Figure 2-3) are the same ones Katherine placed in her first sandtray. They inform the work with Katherine on many levels. Perhaps they represent responses she might have in trying to resolve her losses. The dragon might be anger; the rabbit might represent running away and not facing the pain; the fish turning in upon itself might inspire her to do inner work. For myself, these animals represent different approaches I might take in working with her. The dragon is confrontation; the feminine rooster would be a balance between active intervention and receptiveness; the crab a sidelong approach, keeping things safely distant in the imaginal realm; while the fish reminds me to be aware of my countertransference and keep doing my own personal work.

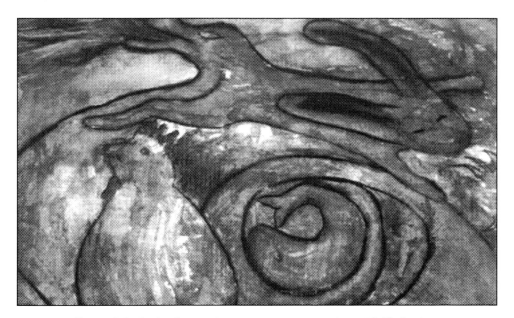

Figure 2-3. Author's painting in response to session with Katherine.

Sandtray with Alzheimer's Patients

An older client with dementia may be overwhelmed by a drawing or painting activity, but often can handle the simplicity of placing objects in the sandtray. The tray itself, a wooden box, provides structure and a clear space within which the client can work. The sand is soothing to the touch and often brings back memories of childhood play and happy times.

For the individual with dementia, the sandtray can be self-soothing, and provide containment, a chance to engage in play. It offers a form of interaction that, for some individuals, is not stressful or disorienting. The concrete quality of the process is attractive to some. However, it is important to remember that Alzheimer's affects each person differently. As seen in the case example below, an individual with Alzheimer's disease might experience a moment of clarity and self-reflection, creating a surprisingly poignant and powerful statement with her sandtray.

Case Example 2: Dora

Dora, age 93 at the time of this work, had end-stage Alzheimer's disease. She was a well-educated woman, a teacher, with a Master's degree in English literature. She had published her memoirs a few years previously. Before her illness progressed, she was playing classical music with friends at least once a week and hosting intellectual discussions that covered everything from literature and politics to existential questions. I was able to do a single session with Dora shortly before she left to live in a nursing home. Her dementia had progressed to the point where this residential site was no longer appropriate for her, because she began to wander off and suffered a series of falls.

Although I did not give Dora a directive in our session beyond simply creating a sandtray, the tray and story fragments she created belong squarely in the realm of fairy tale. The material arose spontaneously, and created an added dimension that taught me a lot about working with this population.

Dora stated that the female figure in her tray is Bába Yagá, surrounded by wild animals. "Bába Yagá can't fight the beasts. They are magical." She repeatedly refered to herself, Dora, as a presence in the tray. When I asked her to point out where she was in the tray, she pointed to the empty space in the corral she had made with three pieces of fence. "I'm here." Knights on horseback surround the corral. "[The knight]'s in my imagination mostly—it'd be nice if he actually showed up and rescued me, took me to my nice, peaceful farm."

Along with the tiger and lion, there is a lamb just outside the corral. "The lamb is close by."

In the midst of her dementia, Dora created a poignant imaginal representation of loss of identity. There seemed to be some confusion about the battle going on, which side was good and which evil. Maybe it was not so much about good and evil, but about internal chaos and struggle. Powerful forces are at work within, over which she had no control. The lamb seemd to be an important image for Dora, and she came closest to identifying with it. She had placed it closest to the empty corral, which she identified as her place in the tray, and spoke of it being "close by." Among all the powerful creatures that populated her sandtray, the one she most nearly identified with was this gentle, helpless lamb. This seemed to reflect her feelings of loss of control in her life. Her reference to the lamb also made me wonder if she was thinking about her death, as this animal is an important symbol in Christianity.

Bába Yagá is the Slavic goddess of life and death. In fairy tales she appears as a witch who eats young children and lives in a hut which turns and dances on hens' feet, surrounded by a fence made of dead men's bones and skulls. She rides through the air on an iron mortar, moving herself forward with a pestle, leaving a trail of death and destruction in her wake. She asks people to do impossible tasks, and if they fail she kills them or keeps them captive (Cotterell, 2000). Did Dora choose this powerful witch to represent Alzheimer's disease, which was eating away her mind?

Estés (1997) recounts the Russian tale of Vasalisa, in which a young woman joins a lineage of wise women as her intuition is awakened. The tasks that Bába Yagá sets for Vasalisa are part of her initiation. Perhaps Dora created a tray about the initiation that occurs at the end of life.

The sandtray and narrative created by Dora include loss and an encounter with a numinous being, touching on parts of Chinen's cycle (1985). The empty corral speaks plainly of loss of self, and the witch might be seen as a representation of Dora's progressive dementia, or as a numinous being. Transformation and resolution do not appear possible in the face of such a destructive force; her story ends with fragmentation. A week after creating this sandtray, Dora moved to a nursing home, due to a series of falls and episodes of wandering away from the site. The momentary clarity that occurred in the session might have been one of the last flickerings of Dora's once-sharp mind and strong spirit.

Painting in response to the session with Dora (Figure 2-4) was quite intense and emotional for me. The figure of Bába Yagá stayed with me after the session, and I knew before entering the studio that she would be the central image in the work. I painted frenetically, with an urgency I rarely experience in the art-making process. I used my hands to apply the paint directly on the paper, rubbing and scratching at its surface. After completing the first piece, the following writing emerged:

> Faceless Enemy: I am darkness. I am your biggest fear and your greatest resource. Rich and fertile. Dark and terrifying. Words cannot even come close or touch this place. A tiny ray of light–a fading star–light from a star that went out already but just took a long time to reach you? Or a last flicker before it's gone forever.
>
> Bába Yagá will eat whatever she can lay her hands on. Your hope. Your promise. Your wishes. She'll eat away until you've just got doubt. Do you dare to look in her mirror, see your soul laid bare? Her house walks and dances on chicken legs, her door is barred by human bones and skulls. Her yard is painted with blood. Sacrifice your ego; give it to her for dinner. Find the warrior woman inside you.

It felt as if Dora and I had been standing on the edge of an endless abyss; for her it was her illness and approaching death, for me sharing this with her was an indescribably powerful and overwhelming experience. At another level all my fears about my worth as a professional and the uncertain future after graduation became activated. After painting a second image, I wrote:

> Terror. Darkness. This box cannot hold me in. I am too powerful. The abyss will engulf all it touches.
>
> No! Facing the abyss is the way to befriend it, harness its power. Turn and face the nightmare monsters. I can use this power for healing. For myself and those who come to work with me. I will not give in to despair.
>
> Surrender.
> Faith.

In this second image, the mirror has transformed into a magnifying glass. Rather than reflecting a terrifying emptiness, forcing us to look into the unknown, Bába Yagá is now an ally who can help us tap into the power of the shadow, teach us the value of the darkness.

For Dora and others with Alzheimer's disease, the sandtray at the very least provides structure and a return to childlike playfulness. In

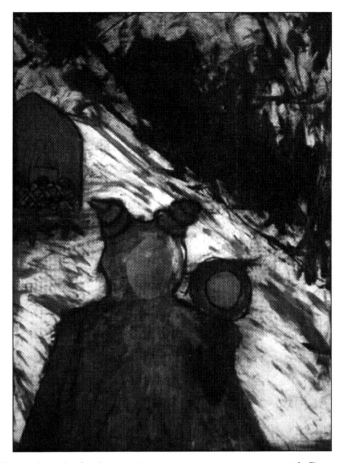

Figure 2-4. Author's painting in response to session with Dora.

this case, Dora's poignant representation of loss of identity suggests to me that a therapeutic experience occurred. She seemed to have had a moment in which she was able to express her fears, her loss, and her struggle in a unique and personal way within the imaginal realm. This probably was not something Dora would be capable of remembering for more than a few minutes, but I believe that the emotional memory of effectiveness, of having made meaning, as well as a feeling of reduced anxiety, stayed with her. I acted as a witness to her process, and perhaps for a moment she was not alone in facing the abyss.

AREAS FOR FURTHER EXPLORATION

Sandtray as Stepping Stone to Other Forms of Creative Expression

As any art therapist who has worked with a geriatric population knows, it can be difficult if not impossible to engage some older adults in creative activity. Many are quite open to the art-making process. However, some older people either feel that they were never artists and have no interest in starting at their age, or that they made art in the past and feel that their art-making days ended when their eyesight began to deteriorate or their hands lost their steadiness. The sandtray can be a way to begin working with symbols, or a road back to creative expression. The ease of producing a finished product with the sandtray figures begins to build the individual's confidence in his/her creative abilities.

For the client who has never made art, experience in the imaginal world can lead to enthusiasm for and trust in one's internal imagery. After several sandtray sessions, the therapist can gradually introduce other art media. For example, a client might be encouraged to use clay to create a simple representation of a figure that is not included in the figure collection. The client might make a simple sketch of a completed sandtray. As the therapeutic relationship grows, the client can become more available to the possibility of using art media to explore the imaginal world, which has become a familiar landscape through the sandtray.

For the artist who feels that he/she cannot make the same kind of art as in the past, new possibilities begin to come into view. Collage is a natural next step from sandtray, as the use of preformed images becomes familiar. As the focus shifts from product to process, from aesthetics to personal meaning, the older adult artist finds new ways to engage in the creative process. In addition to fairy tales, other writing forms can be explored: a dialogue between two figures, a poem, or witness writing, in which the sandtray maker acts as scribe, writing what a figure or whole tray might say.

A painted, drawn, or sculpted image can have multiple layers of meaning for the artist; it might appear in multiple pieces, and evolve as a personal symbol. In the same way, a particular figure can appear in numerous sandtrays over time, and take on highly personal meaning for the tray maker. This easily accessible process opens a door for one to become familiar with his or her own visual language and symbols.

As one begins to trust his or her visual language, drawing or painting becomes far less of a formidable or unattainable prospect. The relationship between the art therapist and the client grows through the sandtray work, and supports further steps toward self-expression. The client experiences what it is like to speak in this often foreign language with relative ease, and the art therapist teaches the client how to interact with and talk about images.

SANDTRAY AS ASSESSMENT TOOL

The sandtray provides a format for comparison of different people's mental states, and so becomes an assessment tool and a rich environment for gaining a glimpse into the landscape of the minds of elders. A tray created by one person with Alzheimer's disease might look different from another suffering from the same illness, but both create the impression for me of fragmentation, a feeling of being lost. Seeing a mind reflected in the sandtray is a powerful and unforgettable experience.

Doing a weekly sandtray session with an individual with dementia can be a way to track changes in mental state and appropriate changes in care might be made. It is important, however, to note that one session may not accurately reflect the individual's overall level of functioning, as he/she may experience fluctuation in the course of the day or week.

What would a Diagnostic Drawing Series (Cohen, Mills & Kijak, 1994) be like if done with a sandtray? The art therapist might ask an individual to complete three trays, starting with an open tray, then a tray depicting a peaceful place, and finally a tray depicting feelings. This is just one possible sandtray assessment to explore. What about a bridge assessment, in which the client would be asked to create a tray using a bridge and any other objects he or she chooses?

SUMMARY

As a nonthreatening format for creative expression, the sandtray meets much lower resistance with the older adult population than art productions requiring greater initiative and self-direction. It can be used as a bridge to work with other media. Weinrib (1983) states that the fact that sandtray work is an active process is especially effective with people who feel powerless and/or hopeless. With an elderly population, moving into action can foster creativity, which in turn feeds one's self image and boosts confidence. There is a high likelihood of success and satisfaction with the sandtray product; therefore the medium supports even the most tentative steps toward creative expression.

The later years of one's life have the potential to be an incredibly creative and fruitful time (Schexnaydre, 1993). We, as art therapists, can use the sandtray to tap into this potential and facilitate an older person's entry or reentry into the imaginal world. Sandtray is effective in the life review process, in addressing developmental issues of aging, and as an assessment tool. It is accessible for older adults with a wide variety of challenges and needs, and offers many levels of reward and satisfaction.

REFERENCES

Bettelheim, B. (1977). *The uses of enchantment: The meaning and importance of fairy tales.* New York: Vintage Books.

Caprio, B. (1993). The sand tray and art therapy. In E. Virshup (Ed.), *California art therapy trends.* Chicago: Magnolia Street Publishers.

Chevalier, J., & Gheerbrant, A. (1996). *The Penguin dictionary of symbols.* New York: Penguin Books.

Chinen, A. (1985). Fairy tales and transpersonal development in later life. *The Journal of Transpersonal Psychology, 17,* 99-119.

Cohen, B., Mills, A., & Kijak, A. (1994). An introduction to the Diagnostic Drawing Series: A standardized tool for diagnostic and clinical use. *Art Therapy: Journal of the American Art Therapy Association, 11,* 105-110.

Cotterell, A. (Ed.) (2000). *Encyclopedia of world mythology.* London: Parragon.

Erikson, E., Erikson, J., & Kivnick, H. (1986). *Vital involvement in old age.* New York: W.W. Norton & Company.

Estés, C. (1997). *Women who run with the wolves.* New York: Ballantine Books.

Schexnaydre, C. (1993). The life review scrapbook technique with the elderly. In E. Virshup (Ed.), *California art therapy trends* (pp.317-332). Chicago, Magnolia Street Publishers.

Tennessen, J., & Strand, D. (1998). A comparative analysis of directed sandplay therapy and principles of Ericksonian psychology. *The Arts in Psychotherapy, 25,* 109-114.

Weinrib, E. (1983). *Images of the self: The sandplay therapy process.* Boston: Sigo Press.

Chapter 3

LIFEBOOKS WITH OLDER ADULTS: MAKING MEMORIES LAST

REBECCA C. PERRY MAGNIANT

As a discipline, art therapy is particularly useful for those who have difficulties expressing themselves with words, due to the mainly nonverbal processes involved. This is one reason why it is useful in working with older adults, especially those with cognitive impairments or brain damage that can impede their verbal abilities. In addition, it seems that people who were born in the early part of the last century have little faith in "talk therapy" and sometimes even less in therapists. The use of art in the process of therapy can help distance the problem, feeling, or memory, put it on the paper, and let the metaphor of the artwork communicate. Working with older adults, I often found that by bringing art into the realm of a session, the clients seemed to forget that it was part of the therapy. The art would allow them to open up in ways that they could not or would not otherwise. Additionally, making art can offer a tangible sense of accomplishment and a visual reminder of work that has been done in sessions. It can also offer a common goal for a group to rally around. And, most importantly, it can say things that words cannot.

With older adults, the goals of working in art therapy are varied. Long-term art therapy can be used to calm someone with anxiety, bring relief from depression, tap into undamaged parts of the brain in an Alzheimer's patient, or help someone grieve. Other goals in working with this population include: increasing self-esteem to focus on the positive abilities of a client; promoting creativity to validate his/her strengths; providing cognitive and physical stimulation; evaluating to assess changes in behavior, ability to follow directions, or make sense of a task; and encouraging social interaction and the establishment of relationships.

This chapter will focus on the use of lifebooks, a technique developed in connection with the life review processes I found naturally occurring with some of my clients. The technique and goals for utilizing this approach will be described, followed by a case study of a lifebook with an older adult client in long-term art therapy.

THE FACILITY

The work described in this chapter was done while I worked at a Continuing Care Retirement Facility (CCRC), a 12-story building that encompasses several levels of care, including a nursing care floor, assisted living, and independent apartments. Clients at the 500-person facility often moved into apartments, transitioning to higher levels of care when needed. It was also not uncommon to find a wife still living in her apartment, while her husband was on the nursing care floor receiving long-term care for dementia or rehabilitation for a broken hip. The clients at the facility, located in the suburbs of a major metropolitan area, were 65 years old and up, mainly middle to upper class, and, for the most part, Caucasian. Clients were always referred to by their family name, out of respect; names in this paper have been changed to protect privacy.

WORKING WITH LIFEBOOKS

The Life Review Process

The lifebook technique described in this chapter was developed to capture the rich verbalizations that accompanied the pictures made by the older adults I was working with. The life review process, described by Bergland (1982) as an ". . . opportunity to integrate thoughts and feelings and consolidate a sense of self" (p. 121), is especially important for people who are nearing the final stages of life. With more time for introspection, the retirement years may be the first time they have had to explore the issues in their lives. Older adults may also have a resurgence of unresolved conflicts and repressed memories at the end of their life. They are suddenly faced with more time in their daily routine to sit and think, and begin to reevaluate issues that they have had for years. The life review process can help to ". . . resolve, reorganize, and reintegrate what is troubling or preoccupying him[/her]" (Lewis & Butler, 1974, p. 165). My impetus to try the technique with lifebook clients was that I wanted to give them order and structure for these thoughts and feelings in a meaningful and lasting way.

Having this defined structure and goal of completing a book charged my clients with a sense of importance and pride. Other positive benefits of life review include a increase in self-esteem, noted in the clients I worked with, as it has been noted by others studying the life review process (Bergland, 1982; Dewdney, 1973; Priefer & Gambert, 1984). For my clients, the lifebooks became both a source of pleasure and pride, a means for self-exploration and catharsis.

Using a spiral-bound drawing pad as their lifebook, the clients illustrated their life stories as they spoke about them. They began to reflect on early-life memories, often the most vividly remembered by older adults as long-term memories have had more time to connect to varied locations in the cortex, making them more easily recalled (Begley, Springen, Katz, Hager, & Jones, 1986). For some, it became a way to reconcile past conflicts and bring up concealed feelings that had been held inside for decades. For others, the lifebook was a way to proudly detail a lengthy career or specific period in his/her life. For all, the life review process presents a tangible way in which to construct ". . . the valuable contributions they have made to their family, their community, and the world" (Drake, 1988, p. 2).

By providing a framework within which to work, older adults using this technique honored the events in their lives, and gained a new sense of place in the later stages of life. They reflected on the past, the present, and what they might like to do in the near future, during this final stage of their life. My clients were aware of the legacy they wanted to leave behind, and these books helped them to achieve this goal.

THE TECHNIQUE

The technique consisted of an inexpensive spiral-bound white draw-ing pad, used as a book. Every week, the client would come up with a memory to depict using pastels, markers, paint, or collage. To some clients familiar with working in mandalas (the Sanskrit word for "cir-cle"), I would offer to draw a circle on the page as a container in which to get started. As the client drew, I would take notes about what he/she said about his/her work. Then I would type up his/her thoughts or "story," bring the typewritten copy back for the next session, and we would put the text alongside the picture, usually on the blank page preceding the picture. (Of course, if able, the client could write the text him/herself, but my clients were either concerned about their pen-manship or lacked the stamina to write after finishing the artwork.)

At the beginning of each session, we would briefly flip through all of the previous pictures. This served to help the client to regain mem-ory over events long past, reorient him/her to the task, and help pro-vide a context in which to find subject matter for the next picture. As the last step, after the desired amount of pages was completed, the client would decide the title of the book and design the cover. (The beauty of a spiral notebook being that if the book was finished but blank pages remained, they could easily be torn out.) I found that lam-inating the cover illustration and then gluing it to the cover of the sketchbook was both visually attractive as well as durable. The client was given his/her book to keep and I made sure, with the client's per-mission, to tell any visiting family members about it, so that the com-pleted project could be shared with them.

Goals and Issues Supported by the Lifebook Technique

One of the first lessons I learned from my supervisor and mentor in the field is that one should keep in mind that older adults have the same issues that younger people do—they have just had them for longer. It might seem strange that a 92-year-old great-grandmother could have issues about her long-dead mother, but all manner of unre-solved issues can resurface when we begin to explore them. Issues can be mammoth or minute, and the lifebooks seemed to bring out a large variety. All of us could make a lifebook about our whole lives, or a period of transition in our lives. However, as people age, and especially as they face the end of their lives, the realization that their days are measured becomes quite real. Older adults begin to think about their lives, putting things into perspective. While some may be content with the paths that their lives have taken, others may realize that they have quite a lot of work to do before they can die with peace.

While there are many techniques and ways of working in art therapy with older adults, I found the lifebooks to be especially successful for certain clients. The following is a list of issues that could be supported by and/or explored with the use of the lifebook technique.

Grief and Loss Issues

Grief can be experienced on many levels–physical, psychological, social, spiritual–and can be a devastating process, whether expected or sudden. Grief may be over subjects as varied as the loss of a person, such as a spouse, or something tangible, such as a home. The grief felt over the loss of someone close can also be accompanied by fear of one's own impending death. Losses seem to accumulate during this period of life, and the lifebook can become a place to honor people and memories.

Life Review Using Early Memories

The following quote by Lewis and Butler (1974) summarizes the process of life review quite nicely. "Life review is seen as a universal mental process brought about by the realization of approaching dissolution and death. It marks the lives of all older persons in some manner as their myths of invulnerability or immortality give way and death begins to be viewed as an imminent personal reality. The life review is characterized by the progressive return to consciousness of past experiences and, particularly, the resurgence of unresolved conflicts" (p. 165). Lifebooks can help a person structure these thoughts, putting them out of the mind and onto the paper.

Supporting Transitions and Transfer Trauma

Transfer trauma is defined as the "physical, mental, and emotional changes which occur when moved from one place to another"

(Virginia Geriatric Education Center, n.d.). With older adults, this can be a move into a nursing home, a move in with one's children, or even a move to another level of care within a facility. This process can be very traumatic—imagine giving up your home of 50 years after you had just lost your spouse. Related to transfer trauma are issues of dignity, dependency, lack of privacy, lack of power, loss of dreams, anger, and depression. The lifebook can help a person maintain some sense of self when everything else is changing, and provide a container for the issues related to transfer trauma.

Promoting Self-Expression, Creativity, and Self-Esteem

Using one's own memories can be a great self-esteem booster, especially at a time when one might be having more trouble remembering. As you age, your long-term memory is often still intact, even if you are suffering from dementia or other memory loss. The lifebook is a great way to stimulate memories, validate one's personal history, enjoy a sense of competence from creating a "book," and validate a person's current strengths. Illustrating one's own life story is a very personal way to express who one was and is.

Leaving a Tangible Legacy

Spaniol (1997) discusses leaving a legacy through one's artwork, and a lifebook is a tangible, memorable way to do this. It can be a conversation starter for families when their older adult is still alive, and a keepsake when they are gone. I found that many of the little stories, things that you would not necessarily tell your children or grandchildren, would come out in the life review process. By capturing them in a lifebook, they were sure to be passed on to future generations.

WORKING WITH MRS. BLOOM

Mrs. Bloom was a 95-year-old widow and had been on the health care unit of the facility for over a year when she started art therapy, although she had spent some time before that in assisted living. Mrs. Bloom grew up in the sunny South, becoming a physical education teacher and spending as much time as she could at the ocean before marrying a doctor and moving up north. When I met her, she did not have the ability to get outside much, never got near the ocean, and could only exercise from the confines of her wheelchair. Mrs. Bloom was referred to art therapy because of her depression and early dementia. The nurses were concerned that the days where she would pack up her belongings to "go home" (part of her confusion) might someday lead her outside of the building alone, which was an obvious safety issue.

While her first sessions in art therapy produced crude, unexpressive imagery, her later imagery brought out a lifetime of memories, relived and revealed through her art. Through our weekly sessions, she warmed up to me and to the art process. The more that she began to trust the process, the more the memories began to pour out. Even the simplest marks on the page (usually in chalk pastel or marker) would get her talking about her life stories. Seeing how much her stories meant to her and how she longed to share them, I asked her if she wanted to start a lifebook, where she would draw or paint a piece of her past every week in art therapy sessions. For this project, we used a blank, spiral bound 11″ x 14″ drawing pad, to which we would later add a laminated cover.

Early childhood memories, usually the most vividly remembered by this population, held special importance, and became a way to resolve past conflicts and bring up concealed feelings that she had held inside for decades. She completed this lifebook during our sessions together and then created a second one, adding one or two pictures a week. The pictures I describe below are in the order that she did them, although other pictures may have been done in-between.

Her Lifebook

Mrs. Bloom started her lifebook with stories of her day-to-day life as a girl. Some were more rich than others—like the time she and her parents went for a walk with one of her neighbor friends and the friend fell into a huge hole in the ground as she tried to pick flowers. After she was rescued, Mrs. Bloom witnessed her friend being beaten for getting dirty, a fact that seemed to startle a young Mrs. Bloom, as her parents did not believe in corporal punishment. The picture itself depicted a tree in the center, with a sloping hill with a large hole in it. This was the first time Mrs. Bloom had drawn a tree, which would mark many pictures after this one.

Pictures that followed this one depicted a tree in the schoolyard that she had played around and her schoolhouse. The tree was now ever present in her work, but always a bit different; for her, it seemed to be a symbol of her youth and her fond memories of it. Several stories also told of how Mrs. Bloom always managed to make something good out of situations that were unpleasant.

Throughout the beginning weeks of the lifebook, Mrs. Bloom's trust in me and trust in the art therapy process began to grow. She consistently remembered my name and associated me with art, although she often got other things confused, and usually thought me to be her "art teacher," as if she was still a child.

Then, for several sessions, Mrs. Bloom created images of stereotypical flowers that seemed to show her lack of drive, and perhaps her reluctance in opening up further. The nurses reported that she had been depressed lately. She confided in me, one day when making a picture of pink flowers, that she often told people that she wanted to jump out of the window, but she never really would because she was afraid of heights. Sometimes we would talk a bit and an idea for an image would pop up; other times, I would bring up the season or the month to see if it triggered any memories for her. There were also times when nothing seemed to spontaneously come forward, and I would offer a collage picture or a figure to help her get started. Pictures that followed in the subsequent weeks marked the change of seasons—one about pumpkins for Halloween, another about fall trees.

In a subsequent session, she was stumped about what to draw. I decided to offer her an image stimulus to place in a drawing, hoping to elicit a more personal response. I asked Mrs. Bloom to pick one of five predrawn figures to include in a setting. She picked a figure in profile, seated, with hands around its knees. Then she selected an orange piece of paper to work on, which we later glued into the book. She placed the figure on the left-hand side of the page, and drew a small lake next to it, so it was sitting on the banks of the lake. She said that the figure had just gotten through swimming and was cold. I then asked her to complete a few Gestalt phrases about her work. By ". . . personifying elements in your artwork and using them to describe your own experiences and perceptions," Gestalt phrases can help one go deeper into the metaphor of the page (Malchiodi, 1998, p. 229). The parts in italics are what I provided her with, and this is the result:

I am near the ocean.
I want to swim, but it's chilly.
I will try a little later.
I feel like swimming, but I don't want to be cold.
I need a little more sunshine.
I wish I were not alone here.
I secretly want to see my boyfriend.
Never refer to me as a vulgar person with no clothes on.

To me, these few, simple sentences poignantly represented her need for sunshine, companionship, and the feel of the water. She spoke more about her love for swimming, skinny-dipping with her husband, and the sadness she felt about not being able to swim any more. I wondered if the last sentence in this Gestalt was a reference to always being taken care of by nurses and losing the ability to care for herself, being both literally and figuratively "naked." It seemed that her issues were becoming clearer, yet they remained in the safety of the figure in the picture, and in the metaphor of the page.

Several weeks later, we had begun to build a strong therapeutic alliance in our sessions. Mrs. Bloom now spoke more openly about the feelings behind the memories brought up by the art making. On this day, she chose a predrawn image of a female form to use to start her picture. She glued it into her book and then filled it in with color; a story then arose as she was coloring the image (see Figure 3-1).

As she described it, this image is a picture of Mrs. Bloom herself at age 14, in a blue party dress. After making this picture, she revealed that throughout her life she had thought (according to her, along with everyone else) that her sister was the prettier one of the two sisters, and had therefore always deserved the prettier dresses. In making this blue party dress, and finally giving *herself* the prettiest dress, Mrs. Bloom let out some of the anger she had repressed over this lifelong jealousy, telling me a secret that she had "never told anyone before." She was also opening up to the possibilities of art therapy, and became more eager to come to our sessions each week.

In the weeks following the party dress picture, her images alternated between her as an adult, ice-skating with her husband, and her as a

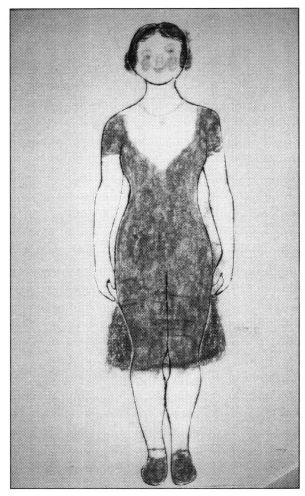

Figure 3-1. "Blue Party Dress"

child, having a snowball fight. The art process seemed to take her to a different place, and at times in her dementia, she would almost act as a young girl, even as she was approaching 100. After one of her sons had come to visit, she depicted a story about a friend's swimming hole after reminiscing about swimming with her boys when they were young. The young girl whose swimming hole it was had been a friend, and as a girl Mrs. Bloom happened to be nearby when the girl was killed in an automobile accident. As this seemed to be her first experience with death, Mrs. Bloom remembered it clearly and was openly moved, perhaps thinking more now about her own approaching death, although not mentioning it.

On this particular day, I found Mrs. Bloom alone in her room, sobbing. She told me that she wanted to leave "this place." I sensed some confusion, as she could not specify where "this place" was. After talking with her, it became apparent that she was longing for home, and felt like she had somehow been separated from her parents. She was confused and bewildered, feeling somehow abandoned but not knowing what to do. Rather than redirecting her, I validated her emotions by suggesting that she make a picture of a place where she would most like to be. She agreed, and came with me to the art therapy room.

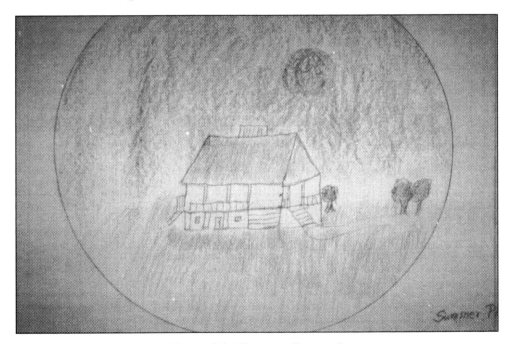

Figure 3-2. "Summer Pleasure"

In the session, she painstakingly constructed a picture of the plantation house shown here, which she described as her grandfather's home (see Figure 3-2). The image of the house was done in pencil and the lower half was shades of green for the grass, the upper half shades of yellow for the sun. When she was finished, she had stopped crying and was visibly calmed and soothed by her image. About the picture, she said that there was a golden sky "because it is the time right before the sun sets." I asked her where she would be if she were in the scene, and she said she would be sitting on the porch, watching the sunset. With this, she seemed to not only want to return to her comfortable, idyllic childhood, but she brought to life the metaphor of the sun-setting on her own life now that she was nearly 100 years old.

In another session, as in previous sessions, Mrs. Bloom was longing for the ocean. She said that she felt most at ease in the water, and that as a girl, she dreamed that she would one day swim the English Channel. Depressed by the fact that "they" would not let her go the pool any longer (due to hip fractures and her poor memory), Mrs. Bloom found a way to immerse herself in the water, almost as if in swimming in heaven, in a collage. When offered a choice of collage images, she chose one of a figure swimming in the midst of a beautiful calming blue. Then she expanded the image by glueing it on a blank page by continuing the water/sky with blue pastel. She titled this picture "Out Swimming in the Clouds" because the image blurred the lines between water and sky. To Mrs. Bloom, swimming under or in the sky seemed to blend her most favorite elements together—her love of the outdoors and her love of the water.

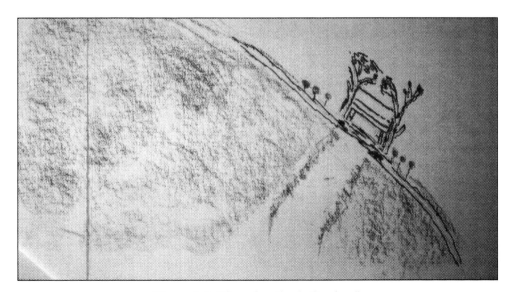

Figure 3-3. "Grandmother's Garden."

This garden was made for grandmother. She worked on it some when she was younger, but stopped when she got older. I think old people gave up earlier in those days, and were pampered by their family. Grandmother sat in her window and looked across the lawn to her garden. . .there were paths going through it with a bench in the bottom path.

On this day, Mrs. Bloom speaks as if she is a young girl and I am her "art teacher." The artwork brings her back to her childhood more often than not now, and she is often taken back into her youth for part of the session. The memory seems to envelops her and allows her to feel what she did back then, if only for a fleeting moment or two.

The image depicts a bench on a hill, with a tree on either side and pink flowers next to the trees. This picture seems to speak to Mrs. Bloom's grief over not being with her family in her old age, and perhaps thinking about a place for her final rest, in a garden near a bench. It may also speak to a sense of loneliness, as she is in a facility, not with her family "pampering" her in her old age. Through the symbolic language of the artwork, we continued to speak, about the nearing end of her life. Thinking back to her grandmother and mother, Mrs. Bloom tried to make sense of where she was now, in relation to where they were at the ends of their lives. Talking about her grandmother had somehow brought her back to present time, and the realization of her current age—an ounce of regret and longing for her own garden, mixed with the proud feeling of having not "given up" and being an active, rather than passive gardener in her own life. (Even then, at 97, she continued to have a window garden in her room.)

A few weeks after she had told me about her grandfather's plantation, she spontaneously drew a small vase of flowers in the lower half of a mandala and wrote this poem to her parents and sister Clara. It said:

Mother, Dad, and Clara
I love you very much
You are in my heart and memories
And I wish they could come true.
Flower bright bring out a dream
Of loved ones far and near
I loved you so, and wish to go
To be with you all the time.

Her thoughts about death and loneliness were apparent in this short poem, as was her sense of being the only one left in the family and

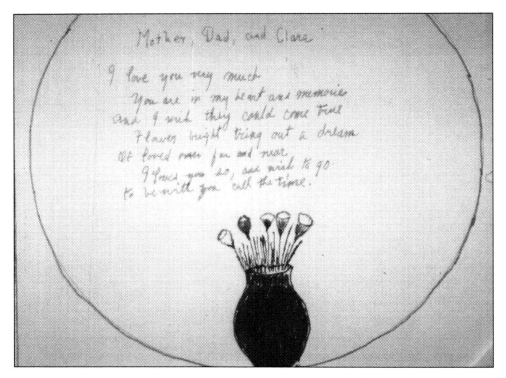

Figure 3-4. Untitled (Mandala and poem).

wishing to go wherever they were. Although this was not the last image in her lifebook, and she created another lifebook after this one, it was one of the most poignant images and truly telling about her emotional state.

For two years after the lifebooks, Mrs. Bloom continued to work in both individual and group art therapy. In individual sessions, she received one-on-one attention, an element that seems to be missing in most nursing home environments. She also got an avid listener, an "art teacher," a therapist, and a way to put into perspective all the things that go along with being alive for almost a century. During our work together, I received fewer calls from the nursing staff asking me to come and work with her when she was found crying in her room. She recognized the art process as something special, where she could share whatever was on her mind that day, and feel validated about it. Her sons cherished her work, and were proud of their mother's accomplishments in art therapy.

DISCUSSION

Although this chapter focused on the use of the lifebooks with individual clients, the technique could easily be applied to a group setting. Group sessions offer clients a different point of view, in that they see their peers in the same life struggles. Many are tickled about becoming an artist in their eighties or nineties, and most seem grateful for a safe forum in which to discuss the emotions and thoughts of everyday life.

Additionally, the technique could be changed to make a lifeline instead of a lifebook, with the whole group working on individual lifelines or on the same mural of their lives intertwined together (Bergland, 1982). Bergland (1982) suggests combining elements of social/world history along with one's personal history in order to give group members perspective into how outside forces and world events may have shaped their lives.

Lifebooks could also be successfully used with other populations and/or age groups, focusing on a similar topic or a certain period of time, such as stories of one's adolescence or a becoming a parent for the first time.

CONCLUSION

Remember this one thing, said Badger. The stories people tell have a way of taking care of them. If stories come to you, care for them. And learn to give them away where they are needed. Sometimes a person needs a story more than food to stay alive. That is why we put these stories in each other's memory. This is how people care for themselves. (Lopez, 1990, p. 60)

Working with older adults in art therapy gives both the client and the therapist the power to collect, cherish, and record the stories of one's life alongside the imagery of it. Lifebooks are a simple and effective way of "taking care" of the stories one is told. As the quote above states, sometimes a person needs a story more that food, and alongside my clients, I found the stories of life to be very nourishing indeed.

REFERENCES

Begley, S., Springen, K., Katz, S., Hager, M., & Jones, E. (1986, September 29). Memory: Science achieves important new insights into the mother of the muses. *Newsweek*, 48-54.

Bergland, C. (1982). The life review process in geriatric art therapy: A pilot study. *The Arts in Psychotherapy, 9*, 121-130.

Dewdney, I. (1973). An art therapy program for geriatric patients. *American Journal of Art Therapy, 12*, 249-254.

Drake, M. (1988, September). Art media with aging adults: Views from near the finish line. *Gerontology, 11* (3), 1-4.

Lewis, M. F., & Butler, R. N. (1974). Life-review therapy: Putting memories to work in individuals and group psychotherapy. *Geriatrics 29*: 165-173.

Lopez, B. (1990). *Crow and Weasel.* San Francisco: North Point Press.

Malchidoi, C. A. (1998). *The art therapy sourcebook.* Los Angeles: Lowell House.

Priefer, B. A., & Gambert, S. R. (1984). Reminiscence and life review in the elderly. *Psychiatric Medicine 2*(1), 91-100.

Spaniol, S. (1997). Guest Editorial-Art therapy with older adults: Challenging myths, building competencies. *Art Therapy: Journal of the American Art Therapy Association, 14*(3), 158-160.

Virginia Geriatric Education Center (n.d.). *Transfer trauma and bereavement.* Training presented at Virginia Commonwealth University, Richmond, VA.

Chapter 4

FOSTERING WELL-BEING AND COMMUNITY IN A CONTINUING CARE SETTING: THE GEORGE DERBY CENTRE ARTWORKS PROGRAM

Pamela J. Brett-MacLean and Marilyn M. Magid

I have wanted to be an artist my entire life and what I was looking for was the feeling. When I came here I was able to get the feeling to let the emotions wash over me." Gerry Garant (Resident, George Derby Centre)

A visit to the Artworks studio provides one with a collage impression: warm welcome, laughter, patient attention, excitement, wild creative visions, simple satisfaction, a quiet absorption, attending to the setting down of a line or dab of colour, just so, sometimes a sense of confusion, and at times frustration. The residents sometimes work together, but most often work alone in the presence of one another in this expansive shared studio space. The art instructors, work along with them. There is a swirl of energy that connects us all. The tender, courageous, often stilling, visual and sculptural creations of the residents call forth a quickening of creative energy that connects all of us, as we work side by side, sharing our visions, our experiences, our stories. Even in the quieter moments, there is always, somehow, an aliveness; an awareness of not yet known, known only in the coming - wild, beautiful arresting, surprising images coming into being. It is this artistic and creative expression that enlivens the community within this continuing care facility.

69

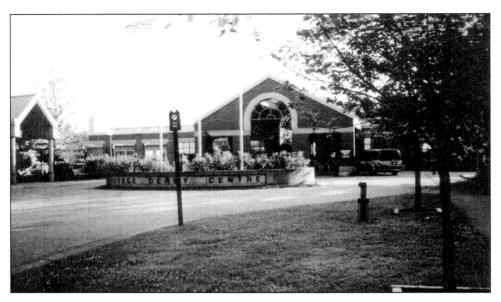

Figure 4-1. The George Derby Centre.

INTRODUCTION

This chapter describes the Artworks Studio program, a well-established arts program for aging war veterans residing at the George Derby Centre in Burnaby, British Columbia, Canada (see Figure 4-1). The chapter begins with a description of the Artworks program, including its orientation and value commitments, program components, participants, and staff. In addition to various creative arts activities, we describe adaptations that have been introduced to facilitate residents' continuing involvement in the program over time, as they experience impaired health, increased frailty, and/or disability. Throughout this chapter, we will illustrate ways in which art making contributes to a sense of well-being, connection, and community, within an institutional care setting and beyond, as veteran residents experience and share their art making with others. We have also included some narratives that may provide a starting point in articulating the tender and elegant, robust and vital potency of the arts in everyday life at a residential care facility. This is done by providing some of the stories residents, family members, and staff at the George Derby Centre have shared in relation to their experience of the Artworks Studio.

GEORGE DERBY CENTRE AND THE ARTWORKS STUDIO

George Derby Centre[1] is a continuing care facility that offers residential care to over 300 elderly Canadian veterans, ranging in age from 75 years old to over 100 years old. The facility originally opened in 1947 to provide physical and occupational therapy, as well as job retraining, to help World War II veterans reintegrate into society following acute care hospitalization and treatment. Over the next 40 years, an increasing number of aging veterans began to receive services from George Derby Centre. In 1988, the Centre relocated from its original barracks location to a new building on adjacent property. Today, as an intermediate care facility, "Derby" serves as both a home and community for elderly Canadian Forces and Merchant Navy veterans who served in World War I, World War II, and the Korean War.[2]

Set in a residential, suburban community near the larger metropolitan area of Vancouver, British Columbia, George Derby Centre occupies a three-level building located on spacious grounds. The front entrance opens to a large foyer that serves to provide a sense of a shared community space. The Centre is organized following an H-shaped design, with a wide range of services situated on the "Main Street" (the connective centre of the building), and four residential units connected to the centre corridor located along the arms of the "H." Along the central corridor, or "Main Street," residents can easily access the multipurpose activity area (also known as the Town Hall), gift shop/ canteen, banking services, dental office, the barber and beauty salon, and the chapel. Many of the Centre's recreational programs are also located along this corridor, including the Music Therapy and Recreation programs, as well as the Artworks Studio, which provides a warm and inviting focal point in the Centre (see

---

1. Continuing care services are designed to assist those individuals who cannot live independently because of ongoing health related problems, but do not require care in an acute or rehabilitation program. Health problems assessed as requiring continuing care are usually of at least three months duration, and are due to a progressive and/or chronic condition. The goal is to provide clients with services appropriate to their long-term functional needs.

2. Other veteran's health care centers in Canada provide residential care and many of these centers offer arts programming. However, the focus, structure, and breadth of programming is unique to each veteran health care center. All of the arts programs are managed independently. A national conference, "Creating a Self Portrait," was held in 1989, to bring staff representatives of 14 sites together to discuss their programs. This chapter provides historical background and descriptive program information that is most relevant to the Artworks Studio Program at the George Derby Centre.

Figure 4-2). In addition to "Main Street" services, residents have direct access to walking paths, gardens, a greenhouse, outdoor courtyards, patios, and gazebos from each of the four residential wings. Along with other members of the multidisciplinary care team, nursing staff provide care to residents who vary across a continuum of required care: those who need more help because of frailty or physical disability, or those who require specialized psychogeriatric care (a Special Care Unit serves veterans experiencing significant cognitive impairment).

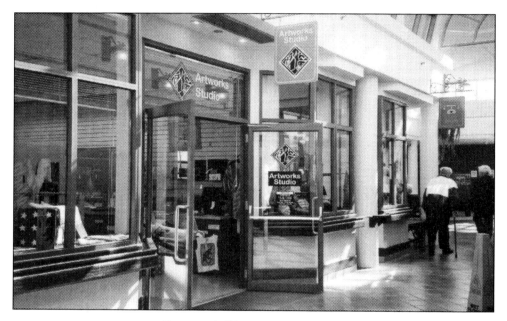

Figure 4-2. The Artworks Studio.

The Artworks Studio is a very active and visible program that offers a comprehensive range of creative arts activities to all of residents of this continuing care facility, both within the Artworks Studio and in each of the residential wings. Similar to the general population, residents of George Derby Centre vary widely in relation to their life contexts and occupational backgrounds. Nevertheless, they share a common background as members of Canadian and Allied Armed Forces serving overseas in armed conflict. Thus, the Artworks Studio program is in many ways unique, in that it is imbued with the memory of wartime service. In addition to physical and cognitive decline experienced by some of the residents, many experience health concerns related to traumatic events experienced during wartime. Further, since most of the residents are male[3], few have been exposed to creative arts and crafts activities, compared to the large percentage of their women peers who have been involved in creative pursuits over the course of their lifetimes. For most male residents who participate, the Artworks program provides them with their first experiences in arts activities. Given this, special attention is given to the process of engaging and maintaining the residents' interest in art making, as well as the development of activities which will attract male participants. Another noteworthy distinction is that the Artworks Studio is one of the most enduring institutional-based arts programs in Canada. The inspiration for the Artworks Studio originated during World War II when Red Cross Society volunteers taught handicrafts to hospitalized soldiers in Newfoundland (Canada), Britain, and on the Continent. Following the war, the continuing need for this program was recognized, for the large numbers of ex-servicemen who required some sort of activity during their long hospital stays. In 1945, the Department of Veteran's Affairs (Canada) and the Canadian Red Cross Society inaugurated a partnership to develop and administer Arts and Crafts programs in veteran's hospitals across Canada.[4] It has continued to evolve and develop in impressive ways as a comprehensive, community-oriented arts program for elderly veterans living in residential care.

Artworks Studio Program Description

Orientation and Value Commitments

The Artworks Studio is based on the belief that art making can enrich life by providing a means of engaging, reflecting on, expressing, and developing life stories, aspirations, and aesthetic visions, while expanding on present interests. Inherent to this view is the notion of artistic expression as a mode of being, providing opportunities for imaginal, expressive, and creative, engagement that enriches

3. Although they are welcomed and honored for their involvement in the war effort, female veterans represent only a very small percentage of the residents at George Derby Centre.

4. This arrangement continued until the mid 1990s when the management of the program was transferred from the Red Cross Society to the individual host facilities in each province. Currently, the Artworks Studio program at George Derby Centre continues to receive federal funding which is used to support a high quality arts program.

one's own life, and the community within which one lives. Ellen Dissanayake (1992), for example, has observed that throughout time and across cultures, art making has fulfilled fundamental needs for human expression, connection, and meaning making. Based on a careful study of the role of art in human evolution, Dissanayake has concluded that art is an inherent and necessary aspect of human behavior. She states that art, "like other common and universal human occupations, and preoccupations such as talking, working, exercising, playing, socializing, learning, loving, and caring should be recognized, encouraged and developed in everyone" (p. 225). John Dewey (1934) the noted American pragmatist philosopher, also argued for the appreciation of art as a potent means for the heightening of one's lived experience through the development of perception and subsequent development of meaning in his text *Art as Experience*. Dewey suggested that through the experience of art, human experience itself becomes expressive, ". . . meanings develop and the self grows through an expanded meaning scape" (Alexander, 1987, p. 4).

More specifically in relation to gerontology, others have also argued for an enhanced valuing of the arts in later life, both in terms of its therapeutic value and *as a part of life*. Weisburg and Wilder (2001) quote the late Dr. Robert A. Famighetti, Director of the Gerontology Centre at Kean University of New Jersey, as saying:

> We, as professionals in the field of gerontology, often neglect to realize the other perhaps more important values of the arts with older adults. For example, the arts can become the language of the aged, a language created over the course of a person's life. The arts can speak for all an older person has been, is, and can continue to become. As an expression of humanity, they are an inseparable tenet in the lives of older persons. Unfortunately, this has been a relatively unknown and neglected quality in the human services system which primarily focuses on the material needs of the aging. The creative arts can provide meaning as the link between the aging human and a society that needs to listen and understand. (p. 23)

As the George Derby Artworks Studio program has evolved over time, it has expanded to realize a number of significant opportunities for experiencing the benefits of art making. Opportunities for creative expression are provided to residents through a variety of art and craft projects that are designed to: (1) promote an aesthetic awareness of, appreciation of, and connection with things in the world beyond the self (e.g., nature, others, stories, materials, aesthetic form); (2) develop skills and/or mastery in a wide range of art and craft techniques; and (3) provide opportunities for residents to experience the creative process. As Eisner (1972) has stated, the "imaginative transformation of feeling, image or idea into some material . . . such that the material becomes a medium of expression" (p. 156). The program also fosters opportunities for relating and connecting with others (such as staff members, family, and friends) throughout the art-making process, including public display of completed artworks both within the Centre and in the local community.

As they are aware that very few of the residents have experience with art making during earlier periods of their life, Artworks Studio instructors are sensitive to the concerns many residents have about becoming involved in the program. Given this, program instructors provide friendly encouragement and support to residents. Ongoing, informal assessment of a resident's abilities and interests guides the supportive efforts of art instructor staff. Following assessment of residents' physical and cognitive abilities, interests, and level of motivation, an art instructor will usually suggest a specific art activity that the resident may want to take on as their initial art project, although residents have the final decision about which projects they would like to undertake. Residents build on their experience over time, exploring different approaches to creative expression as they gain technical skills. (See the later section on "Staff and Structural Support" for additional details regarding the instructional support provided to residents.)

Program Components

To encourage ongoing participation and enjoyment of the program, art instructor staff and volunteers endeavor to: (1) provide a safe environment in which to work and experience creative growth; (2) provide friendly encouragement that serves to support, motivate, and challenge residents through the process of art making; and (3) foster opportunities for social interaction and recognition of the residents' creative efforts.

A variety of means are used to ensure residents are aware of and feel personally invited to become involved in the Artworks Studio program. As noted earlier, the Artworks Studio is situated in a prominent location in the main foyer of George Derby Centre. Two sets of double glass doors which open to the "Main Street" serve to invite participants into the bright and lively workshop environment. Large bay window displays of residents' artwork also offer an appealing invitation to curious passersby. In addition, brochures describing the program are included in welcome packages when residents and their family members are given a orientation tour of the facility. Classes and special workshops are offered throughout the center to introduce new residents to the program. Art instructor staff also approach individual residents and invite them to visit and tour the Artworks Studio. Some residents visit the studio with their family members, friends, volunteers, or paid companions.

Instructors will also approach residents who may have previously been involved with the program, and invite them to return to the Artworks Studio to begin or continue working on an individually designed project. Staff will maintain contact to stay in touch with residents who become ill, return from the hospital, or suffer a setback such as a stroke. In these cases, staff will visit often and offer encouragement when the resident is ready to resume his/her creative activities. In cases where the resident's condition does not improve, instructors continue to visit the resident, bringing cards, completed art projects, words of support and caring from everyone, and news from the studio. When a resident dies, a special collection of all of his/her completed art projects are given to his/her family, recognizing the legacy of his/her gift of creative expression. Stories about the significance of art in the life of the resident during their time at George Derby Centre, and how it was valued by families, are often shared with staff during these occasions.

Overall, a wide range of arts-based activities are provided throughout the facility–including Artworks Studio activities, outreach activities, and community programming–to ensure that all of the residents are aware of, and exposed to the creative expression of the community. Indeed, most of the residents are actively involved in art making–in some form–as part of their everyday life as residents of the George Derby Centre.

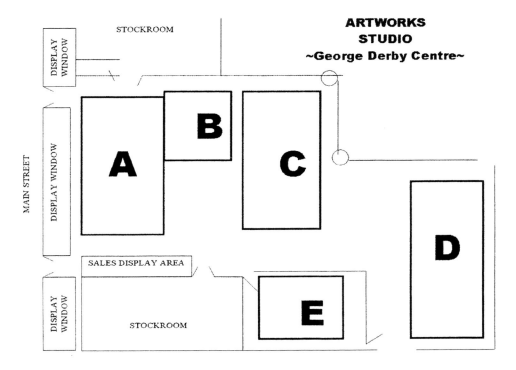

Diagram 4-1. The Artworks Studio Layout.

Artworks Studio Activities

The Artworks Studio is open every day but Sunday. The studio occupies approximately 3,000 square feet of space and is apportioned into a number of different creative activity areas, including a large weaving area (see Diagram 4-1, area "A") comprised of 14 table looms and eight floor looms, a large warping mill, and layout/cutting station, and sewing machines. Another significant area of the studio is committed to painting (area "B"). Other areas of the studio are devoted to a variety of arts activities such as paper-based arts (drawing, sketching etc.); sculpture-based arts (hand-building clay work, paper maché, etc.); textile arts (including needlework) and woodworking projects (area "C"); ceramics (area "D"); and computer-based art projects ("E").

Individual and group-based art-making activities take place in the Artworks Studio across almost all of these areas throughout the week (see Figure 4-3). Although weaving projects tend to be more individual-focused, other arts projects (painting, paper maché sculpture, etc.) can be completed by individuals working alone, in small groups surrounding a table, or in pairs such as a wife or daughter and a father, a resident and a companion, or a resident and a volunteer visitor. Art instructors are assigned to each of these areas, and are responsible for greeting the residents and providing support and instruction in an informal and individualized manner through the duration of a resident's visit to the studio.

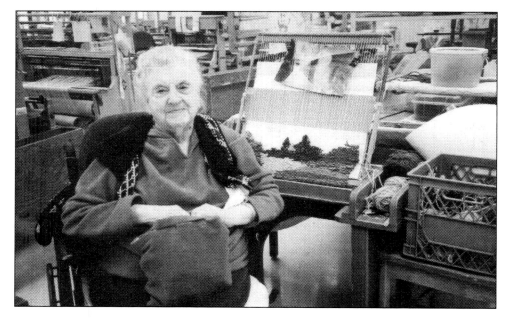

Figure 4-3. Mary MacLean with her tapestry weaving project in the studio.

As residents gain confidence in their skills and abilities, some find the use of a personal notebook particularly helpful in documenting their ideas and creative explorations. These notebooks often include photographs of completed works, as well as drawings of images that have inspired them. In many ways, these notebooks can be considered works of art in themselves. Other residents have brought photographs of their family home, family members, pets, or other evocative images into the workshop to use as inspiration for art projects.

Collaborative "theme-based" workshops are also organized on special occasions in the Artworks Studio. The workshop activity chosen is something everyone can do, and usually involves only one or two steps. Some projects, like creating cards for Christmas or Valentine's Day, allow the residents to take finished articles away with them. Instead of having only a one-day workshop, the Valentine theme has been extended over a longer period to give residents a chance to make heart-shaped articles such as clay pins, wall pieces, candleholders, and lanterns in time for the holiday. Staff and family members often attend these workshops as a social event. Other collaborative projects have involved students working with residents on community arts projects (see section titled "Community Arts Programming"). The range of in-studio arts projects and activities that are supported as part of the Artworks Studio program are described in Table 4-1.

Table 4-1. Examples of Artworks Studio Arts Projects

Studio Area	Examples of Art Projects and Related Activities
A. Weaving	Residents have explored color themes by visiting the botanical gardens and taking photos of the flowers that inspired them. Upon their return to the studio, they have used the photographs to inform their palate for weaving. Residents have also explored their family tartans through a historic tartan pattern book and completed projects using their family colors. Residents who did not have a family tartan made up one for themselves. Sewing machines and a serger are often used to transform fabric into a wide range of finished articles, including placemats, shawls, tea towels, as well as jackets, sweaters, and other garments.
B. Painting (Watercolor, acrylic, and latex paints on canvas, wood, or glass; Fabric painting with dyes)	Depending on an individual resident's needs and interests, painting projects may be designed by the instructors for the resident or may be designed by the residents themselves with support by the instructors. In addition, ready-made articles such as tablecloths, napkins, t-shirts, aprons and umbrellas are also used for a number of painting projects. A popular project involves dabbing a long, white silk scarf tied in small knots with fabric paints (following principles of complementary colour mixing) to create a beautiful pattern.
C.1 Paper-based Arts (Drawing and sketching; collage; stamping, stenciling; printmaking)	Paper-based arts projects are fast, easy, and adaptable to any level of ability. Paper-based arts techniques have been used to create greeting cards, as well as prints, and other decorative works. Personal photographs and greeting cards received from family and friends are often incorporated into these projects.

Table 4-1. Examples of Artworks Studio Arts Projects (continued).

C.1 Paper-based Arts (Drawing and sketching; collage; stamping, stenciling; printmaking)	The small Japanese printing press called a Gocco has provided a simple and effective means of copying two-dimensional images without the need for advanced drawing skills. Images are reproduced with a copier and then transferred onto a small screen using the printing press. No solvents or other special equipment is involved.
C.2 Sculpture-based Arts (Paper maché, Doll-making, Basket-making)	Some of the objects that residents have created using paper maché include human figures, large animals (such as cows and sheep), as well as small fruit and vegetable arrangements. A group of residents were involved in the production of a life-size person with student volunteers from the nearby high school. The figure was called "Mr. Very Special," and he traveled all over the facility with the staff and the students engaging as many people as possible in the "operation." The participants were even given lab coats to extend the metaphor. In the end, Mr. Very Special became a mascot for the Centre. Residents have also collected twigs from the grounds of George Derby Centre to make dolls, doll furniture, and baskets.
C.3 Textile Arts (Needlework or stitchery; Bargello or long stitch embroidery; Off-loom weaving)	Residents' imagery for stitchery varies widely from animals, seasonal ideas such as Christmas stockings, sea or landscapes, and has also included storybook illustrations. Bargello is a long stitch embroidery technique that is designed to cover large areas of canvas, and is easily adapted to varying levels of ability. As each Bargello stitch can cover up to 15 mesh holes, this technique is a good alternative for residents who are no longer able to do small-scale needlepoint. An example of a textile project completed by a group of veterans was a wall hanging with each person stitching a square depicting a favorite memory from childhood. One square captured the image of the family dog while another depicted a rider holding his hat in the air while riding a horse at a rodeo.
C.4 Woodworking (Furniture; toys; game boards and pieces)	Decorative furniture pieces have been created by residents, such as high back chairs with animal images painted on them. Adirondack chairs have been used in a project developed for residents on the psychogeriatric unit. Each person is given one piece of the chair and is invited to paint it according to his/her own stylistic preferences. The colors chosen are primary colors so even though all of the marks vary from person to person, the colors unite the pieces into one whole.

Table 4-1. Examples of Artworks Studio Arts Projects (continued).

C.4 Woodworking (Furniture; toys; game boards and pieces)	A series of game boards was recently completed by a group of residents who painted the wooden boards and made ceramic pieces to go with them. Parcheesi©, Checkers, Chess, and Scrabble© games have all been made in group workshop sessions with participants sitting around a table working on their section. Conversations and reminiscing about games and playing are encouraged and enjoyed by all participants in these sessions.
D. Ceramics (Hand-building, painting bisque ware, slip casting)	Hand-building pottery is popular with many residents interested in exploring either functional pots or creating more elaborate sculpture. The residents take great pleasure in working with malleable clay material and developing their own unique and creative artworks. Many hand-built projects are begun by placing the clay into forms such as bowls or plates to support the object that is being created. Ready-made bisque ware such as teapots, cups, and saucers, etc. is available for residents to paint with commercial glazes and fire. Liquid clay slip is also used for ceramics projects to reduce the cost of materials, since purchasing bisque ware from a supplier is expensive. The clay slip is poured into simple molds, and later painted with commercial glazes and fired.
E. Computer-based Arts	A resident who has a digital camera has used his photographs to create greeting cards, bookmarks, gift enclosures, and calendars using the computer. He has undertaken an ongoing project photographing the grounds of George Derby Centre from all angles in all seasons. It has been suggested that an annual calendar based on residents' photography work be instituted by the Artworks Studio program. Another resident is interested in quotations, poetry, and historic moments in time that are meaningful to him. He develops compositions of these printed narrative excerpts, in conjunction with photo images of his choice. These images are then printed and laminated to form either literary bookmarks or placed in a frame for sale.

Artworks Outreach Activities

Individualized outreach sessions are offered one or two times a week to residents who are sick, recently returned from the hospital, or reluctant to leave their rooms. These art-making sessions provide residents with the opportunity to experience a creative arts project in a quiet, nonthreatening environment. Using a rolling cart, art instructors take materials to a resident's room and spend about ten minutes with him or her (although these sessions may be longer, depending on the resident's interest, stamina, understanding, and enjoyment). Typically, individualized outreach activities will involve small artmaking projects such as painting a silk scarf, printing a card, or using a brush to add color to a wood project. For residents who are unable to leave their room, this is the only connection they have to the Artworks Studio program. Even so, each person who participates in these sessions seems to enjoy the social and creative quality of the activity, however brief it might be.

Group workshop sessions are organized once or twice a week on each of the residential units (see Figure 4-4). As individuals become frail or confused, they often prefer to work on art-based projects in a quiet, familiar setting. Organized group-based workshop sessions also provide an option for residents who may be unwilling to attend the Artworks Studio due to uncertainty about involving themselves in the art process, or committing themselves to a long-term project.

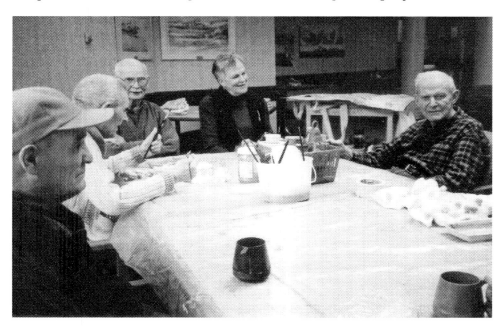

Figure 4-4. Group workshop held on a residential unit.

Group workshop sessions may take place in the dining room or in one of the lounges located in the different residential units. Each session typically lasts an hour. Instructors pack up all the art materials that are required for a specific group project, and travel to different units of the facility inviting the residents to participate in creating a collaborative artwork. Although all residents in attendance are encouraged to participate in some way, they are not required to do so. During the group sessions, residents may come and go as they wish. Some residents choose to simply observe. Art-making projects in these sessions usually involve the creation of easily recognized or familiar objects (fruit arrangements, fish, etc.) using simple arts techniques and use of materials that provide tactile stimulation (painting, paper maché). Projects are designed so that any mark or contribution that a resident makes is viewed as a welcome and valued addition to the overall project. As an example, a group of residents were presented with different pieces of a wooden chair to paint. As each resident completes his piece, a wonderful mélange emerges revealing a unique pattern of color and shapes as the chair is assembled.

As occurs with most of the Artworks Studio Program activities, group workshop sessions foster a time of reminiscence as the residents share stories of the past, as well as discussion of present interests (such as gardening, picnics, carpentry, visits, outings, etc.). These group workshop sessions have proved to be an effective way to support residents in remaining active in the Artworks Studio program during periods of illness and convalescence. In addition, many residents have become involved in activities in the Artworks Studio program because of their experience in workshop sessions on the residential units, and encouragement of family members who learn of the program through these sessions. These sessions have also proved to be a particularly appropriate means of engaging residents on the psychogeriatric unit in creative activity.

Community Arts Programming

Community art projects are another important component of the Artworks program. George Derby Centre residents have enthusiastically contributed to a wide range of fund-raising and community-based artworks activities. Residents have made soup bowls to raise money for the needy. They have also created clay sections for a community totem project that was installed on the grounds of the local City Hall complex. All of these projects have helped to build connections within the larger community.

Intergenerational arts projects involving residents and children from the local elementary and high schools have also been a popular component of the Artworks Studio program. During the school year, students from the high school in the neighborhood volunteer in the studio. They come in pairs to either work with residents to create special art projects, such as a large paper maché animal, or to socialize one-to-one with residents who would benefit from the social contact. "Make and Take" workshops enable residents and youth to work together on a small arts project (such as a painted bookmark or picture frame which can be created in one or two steps). The residents benefit from sharing their art-making skills and experience with the students. In addition, stories are often shared, and understanding and friendship fostered across the generations. The art object that is taken home by the student serves as a reminder of positive feelings of connecting with seniors.

Intergenerational arts projects have also involved connections with the larger community. George Derby Centre residents and students at Cariboo Hill Secondary School were invited by the City of Burnaby to paint banners that were later placed on lampposts on the street between the two facilities. Most recently, residents of George Derby Centre have worked with students from a local elementary school on a project called "The Web of Life in our Neighborhood." Students, residents, and volunteers associated with the George Derby Centre have spent many hours painting and decorating wooden pieces that will soon be installed on the school fence.

Trips to local art gallery shows, country fair competitions, botanical gardens, and other sites are also arranged two or three times a year. These outings are very popular with the residents. These trips provide the basis for discussions and critiques about art and art making, and provide opportunities for sketching ideas that may be used in later art projects. Museum visits, art books, and exhibits of residents' art in the display windows of the Artworks studio (see below) provide an opportunity for participants to actively consider different art forms, and to expand the realm of possibility of their creative expression.

The People Involved in Artworks

Participants

Including Artworks Studio, "outreach" activities, and community arts programming, over 175 of the 300 residents are involved in some aspect of the Artworks Studio program within a one-month period. On any given day, the number of residents who make use of the Artworks Studio space ranges from 30 to 50 residents. There is an ebb and flow to the movement of the participants, which depends on mealtimes as well as on other activities offered in the facility (for example, a musical event or a dance). Although mornings tend to be busier, many of the residents who make regular use of the program attend the program from the moment the program opens in the morning until it closes at the end of the day. Many of the participants in the program consider their involvement in the Artworks program to be as important as any job they used to have, and their daily attendance attests to their commitment to their postretirement vocation.

Although the number of residents involved in the program varies each month, about ten percent have been involved in the program for longer than 20 years, and another ten percent for more than eight years. More recently, with increased emphasis placed on helping veterans stay in their homes longer, involvement in the program involves shorter periods of time than the long periods of involvement of the past. Currently, most residents actively participate in the program for one to five years.

There are many factors involved in the termination or interruption of involvement in the program: death, sickness (including falls and strokes), fatigue and depression, increasing frailty, and cognitive impairment. As described earlier, even when illness or increasing levels of disability and impairment are experienced, Artworks program staff will maintain contact with the resident through outreach activities, and will also introduce adaptations to enable continuing involvement in creative arts experiences (see the following section.)

Residents who regularly participate in the Artworks Studio program include those who are independently mobile, and can make their own way to the studio. Artworks staff, nursing staff, and paid companions assume responsibility for reminding other residents with cognitive impairments to come to the studio for a morning or afternoon session.

Daily records are kept of residents who have participated in the program, as well as those residents that art instructors have visited that day. An effort is made to ensure that all residents who have enjoyed being involved in art projects in the studio are contacted on a regular basis. Artworks Studio staff and others have observed that long-term art practice "brings a kind of inner rhythm and stability that affirms earlier growth and builds confidence for future more ambitious engagements" (London, 1989, p. 111). Given this, Artworks Studio staff work to sustain a resident's involvement in the program, and provide conditions that may enable them to deepen their experience of the possibilities and potentials of creative expression.

Still, a few of the residents elect to enjoy only a passive appreciation of arts programming available through the program. They may not be interested in creating arts and crafts projects but may visit and chat with other residents and art instructor staff working in the Artworks Studio, enjoy artwork displays, and purchase articles for themselves or as gifts for family and friends.

Staff and Instructional Support

Five full-time and four part-time arts instructors staff the Artworks Studio program. Two instructors work in the weaving area with as many as 15 weavers at a time. The rest of the room, which includes 11 large worktables that can each accommodate four to six participants, is covered by five instructors. Many of the instructors involved with the program have degrees or diplomas in the fine arts, art education, or arts and crafts, or are accomplished self-taught artists. All instructors have experience teaching a wide range of art and craft techniques; most have learned to adapt techniques to the needs of residents experiencing physical and cognitive impairments during the time of their involvement with the Artworks Studio program (see the following section). The program is also assisted by four volunteers who participate in the program one day a week for an average of five hours. Volunteers are selected on the basis of evidence of interest in interacting with veterans, knowledge and skills in arts and crafts techniques, and an ongoing commitment to participate on a weekly basis. All staff and volunteers are enthusiastic and energetic, flexible, intuitive, and caring.

As mentioned earlier, a "resident-centered" approach is used to foster technical skill development, as well as refinement of creative expression. Both at an early stage and throughout a resident's involvement in the program, a friendly, informal approach is used to assess residents' functional abilities, including: personal interests and hobbies; past achievements; physical ability (such as strength, dexterity, and mobility); awareness, attention span and tolerance; motivation, initiative, and willingness to participate; and social ability, habits, and preferences (Canadian Red Cross Society, 1989, p. 1). Instructors will also watch for ways of engaging residents who may be more reserved, or not verbally communicative, by making eye contact and encouraging their involvement.

The open, ongoing nature of the program provides residents with an opportunity for developing their technical art-making skills and artistic vision over time. Many residents lack confidence in their art-making abilities, or may be experiencing depression. Given this, art instructors usually suggest that a resident start with a small, relatively simple project that is designed to instill confidence and continuing interest in the program. The instructor will help the resident get started on the project, assist the resident with the project, or simplify the project as needed. The resident's progress on this project is used to establish a benchmark for the resident's level of ability, as well as his/her need for instruction and assistance. To help a resident recognize his/her potential, art instructors provide friendly encouragement and reassurance, and ensure that the resident experiences success at a project that is meaningful or of interest to them.

Technical skills at this early stage may be refined through approximation. For example, copying is often used to facilitate learning. Later projects introduce increasing levels of complexity and mastery of technical skills to help ensure that the work provides the resident with an appropriate level of challenge, and an opportunity for new learning, creative expression, personal enjoyment, and sense of achievement. Participants are encouraged to explore their preferences for particular art forms, subject matter, color selection, and incorporation of personal experiences. Instructors will also help program participants explore different color relations and other expressive aspects of the project.

The management team at George Derby Centre is committed to a multidisciplinary team approach to resident care. Artworks Studio staff work collaboratively with other programs in order to promote effective relationships and communication processes with other staff members, including support staff, nutritionists, kitchen staff, social workers, medical staff, etc. Artworks Studio staff contribute to inter-disciplinary care conferences and care planning, as required. They have also worked with rehabilitation aides, recreation workers, and the music therapist to develop a programming approach that ensures a smooth transition between programs for more confused residents, particularly those on the psychogeriatric unit. For example, a rehabil-itation aide may begin a program for cognitively impaired residents in the dining room, which will be immediately followed by an Artworks Studio workshop. During the last 15 minutes of the workshop, the music therapist may arrive to begin a soft music session that continues until the tables are set for lunch.

Adaptive Techniques

Even as Artworks Studio participants learn technical and expressive art-making skills over time, increasing age and frailty often necessitates ongoing adaptations. Artworks Studio staff have learned that individ-ualized assessment and instruction, alteration of the environment, adaptation of the art-making project, and use of aids can ensure that interesting, challenging, and sophisticated art- making experiences may still be enjoyed by participants. A variety of adaptive tools, including gripping aids, cutting and visual aids, as well as stabilizing aids can be used to enable a resident to continue working on art and crafts projects. For example, a clamp may be used to stabilize a needle-point frame, or use of a pair of pliers can help an individual with use of one hand, or hand tremors, to pull a needle through canvas. However, it is important that adaptations that are introduced are responsive to the needs of program participants, and do not compro-mise the resident's sense of challenge and enjoyment.

Table 4-2 lists a few examples of adaptive techniques that have suc-cessfully been incorporated into the Artworks Studio program. Some key resource references that may be helpful in identifying useful adap-tations and techniques include: *An instructors guide to crafts for special needs* (Canadian Red Cross Society, 1989); *Arts for older adults: An enhancement of life* (Hoffman, 1992); *Training personnel to teach art to older adults living in special care facilities* (Hubalek, 1998); and *A participant observation study of an art class for physically-challenged adults* (Stokrocki, 1998).

Table 4-2. Examples of Adaptive Techniques for Specific Impairments

Project	Materials	Adaptive Technique
Painting for participants with visual impairments	Paint, fabric, brush, wooden frame	A wooden frame is placed on top of a fabric canvas (such as a t-shirt) to create a concrete border for the painter. Directions are provided that describe the frame, and hand-over-hand guiding is used to show the painter the parameters of the section to paint. Color selection and mixing is discussed with a view to creating a pleasing result.
Weaving for wheelchair-bound participants with visual impairments, and use of one hand	Loom, cue cards (attached to the loom, hung in front of the weaver)	A cue card is created with string glued down in the shape of the weaving pattern. If the weaver is using a 1+2, 3+4 pattern, these numbers are glued on the cue card. Each time the weaver changes the shed to the appropriate number, a small clip is moved to the next set of numbers. In this way, the weaver can feel his pattern, as well as his location in the sequence of numbers. The loom levers are placed in a row, so the weaver can feel and count the levers (1, 2, 3, or 4). These levers are adjusted to be accessible from the left or right side so a weaver with the use of only one hand can access the levers on the appropriate side. Loom tables are raised and lowered to accommodate the varying heights of wheelchairs.
Group painting class for residents with impaired cognitive ability and short term memory loss	Ceramic tile, or a piece of fabric; paint or glaze	The project is broken down into small steps, and instructions are provided one step at one time (e.g., 1–"take your brush and put it into the glaze," 2–"place the brush on your piece of ceramic tile"). Instructions are repeated as many times as needed to ensure that everyone understands the process. Everyone benefits from the repetition of instructions without feeling singled out. All participants are encouraged to choose whichever color he wants, and are reassured that all colors and markings are appreciated and considered creative. Participants are also encouraged to discuss ideas, themes, and memories, related to the project.

Narratives

It is difficult to capture the many ways that the Artworks Studio program has impacted the George Derby Centre residents and staff, family and friends, and the larger community. In this section, a number of narratives are presented with a view to fostering an ongoing conversation among policymakers, interdisciplinary health care teams, program planners, and seniors, about the potency of the arts in enhancing life within a residential care community.

Residents

"I have always been a person who loves a challenge. When I came to the Centre because of my cancer, I didn't expect to find a place where I could learn something new. Weaving every day at the Artworks Studio gives me a reason to get out of bed in the morning and helps me take my mind off of my cancer." –Resident, 80 years old, receiving palliative care, weaver involved with the Artworks Studio for 12 months.

"I like to go down to the art room because it is like normal life with coffee, conversation, and freedom." –Resident, 70-year-old female veteran, involved one year.

"I was surprised to find that there would be so much to look forward to learning and experiencing here." –Resident, 85 years old, involved with the Artworks Studio for 15 years.

Family Members, Friends, and Companions

"Looking at the benefits of this program, I feel for the people living in other facilities who don't have such a creative program such as this. The residents are full of pride, happy, and feel useful. One of the residents I know well is respected for his work, and proud to be able to earn his way in the world by selling his weaving. He has stopped worrying so much and it seems to have reduced his mental stress." – Volunteer, (retired principal), one year.

"This place has kept my dad alive. Men of that generation were used to going to work, and coming here kept his hands and mind busy. The staff are some of the most compassionate and caring staff in the whole centre." –Daughter, whose father participated for five years.

"First thing for me is that the program gives a focal point for a visit. My husband has little conversation, so the crafts absorbs the conversations because we talk about colors, shapes, textures, rolling out clay and how pretty things are. This program is like coming to a club for people who like to do things. Afternoon coffee is part of the club and many come in for the social contact. My husband doesn't remember his achievements but for those participants who do, there is a sense of accomplishment and self worth. They are still able to provide, but in a different way. His value in himself was what he could do and since he was no longer able to do things, he has no value. Here, he is busy doing things and has a fairly long period of concentration. Here, he works for 1 1/2 hour session, with tea, three to four times a week. This program is a godsend." –Wife of a resident on the Special Care Unit, four years involvement.

Art Instructor Staff

"I remember a time when the head of Geriatric Medicine took her students on rounds and introduced them to a resident with severe Parkinson's disease. This resident had difficulty controlling his tremors, and was not able to eat or dress independently. The doctor asked the group what they might expect this patient was capable of doing by himself and the response was "very little." Somewhat later that morning, the doctor brought her students to the Artworks Studio where they saw the resident creating a weaving on a 9' x 4' tapestry loom, using a large wooden needle to weave a landscape with no evidence of tremors. The students learned that the resident worked at least three hours every day, five days a week on his weaving. After this session, the students had changed their assumptions about what is possible in spite of severe limitations." –Instructor working with the Artworks Studio program for 20 years.

"In the past, we as instructors were trained to believe that satisfaction for the residents was the end product. Now it's the creative process that is most important. Learning techniques, designing, and having the project evolve is a whole process that is different for each participant." —Instructor, 25 years.

Other George Derby Centre Staff

"One of the best examples of your success are the residents who arrive in our facility unsettled, nervous, unable to sleep, and whose lives are transformed when they find that they enjoy making things. They find a purpose, something they enjoy, and they have a way of giving something back to the people who are important to them." — Registered Nurse, working at the George Derby Centre for 25 years.

Artworks Studio Displays and Exhibits

Prominent display windows of the Artworks Studio, and a window display case in the psychogeriatric unit, provide a means of celebrating the accomplishments of individual or groups of residents. Displays may focus on the breadth and diversity of the residents' creative output or recent artwork projects, including those focused on various seasonal and aesthetic themes. A recent window display included artworks of several residents that were created in honor of the 100th birthday of another resident. Another display highlighted experimental work completed by one resident who was interested in exploring the changes in the appearance of a weaving pattern when a color change is introduced in the weft of a placemat. Artwork is displayed over a two to four-week period to provide residents, staff, family, and other visitors an opportunity to view the displays. Artworks Studio program instructors share their ideas and plan the displays which may showcase a series of projects completed by a resident, or a number of group projects that may have recently been completed. In addition, if a resident has expressed interest in showing his/her work, then a display will be developed to showcase the work.

An annual Artworks Studio Exhibition that showcases the work of all Artworks Studio program participants takes place in the fall, when the studio is transformed into a gallery space over a two-day period (Friday and Saturday). Over 100 visitors attend this exhibit every year. Invites to this annual event include: family, friends, and staff members; residents and staff from other continuing care facilities in the area; and other community members and organizations. Similar to other gallery show openings, the opening of the Annual Exhibit and other special exhibits often involves invitations, advance publicity, a formal reception, and public recognition of the residents' work. Photographs of the residents are displayed along with their artwork, and many residents attend the exhibition and are happy to discuss their work with visitors. Many will also demonstrate different art techniques, and their work on ongoing projects.

Exhibitions and competitions in local venues present the residents with the opportunity to display their work in the larger community, as well as compete for awards with other artisans. Each year, a selection of the residents' artwork is sent to competitions such as the Pacific National Exhibition and Cloverdale Country Fair, where many of the entries (in particular, weaving entries) have won prizes for excellence in their class. Residents' artwork is also exhibited at the local library and community art galleries on a regular basis. Exhibits such as these have provided significant opportunities for public recognition of the residents' creative efforts. The praise and positive attention of others has contributed to the residents' sense of pride in a job well done, and has inspired them to carry on with their own creative pursuits. These experiences have also contributed to the development of significant connections with the larger community. For example, a special exhibit of 20 weaving panels created by residents of the George Derby Centre was organized in collaboration with the Department of Adult Education at Simon Fraser University (in Burnaby, British Columbia). During the opening reception, residents, program staff, and faculty members had an opportunity to meet and discuss the residents' work. The Dean of Education, in addressing those assembled, suggested that although universities and continuing care facilities often exist in isolation from on another, the exhibit had convinced him of the importance of maintaining an ongoing connection with the Artworks Studio program.

Whenever a special community exhibit or event has taken place, photographs or digital recordings of the event are taken to record the event for those who were not able to attend. In this way, other members of the community (including residents' family members and friends) can experience and discuss the event and the creative accomplishments of the veterans.

Artwork Purchase and Sales

Although the Artworks Studio program is offered free of charge to residents, completed artwork is available for sale. Each article is priced to cover the cost of all materials, and residents are offered first choice in purchasing an artwork. If a resident wants to purchase his own work then he pays for those materials. A resident may also decline to purchase a work, preferring that it be put forward for public sale. When this occurs, a small honorarium is added to the cost of materials and the article in place in the gift shop for sale. The honorarium is given to the resident once the article is sold.

Many residents do purchase favorite pieces of artwork to decorate their rooms, or to give as a gift to family or friends. Indeed, many artwork pieces begin with the idea of making them as gifts. For example, one resident, who learned to weave when he was 96, wove a number of *courier de bois* scarves that he later gave to members of his family to celebrate his 100th birthday. Another resident whose father-in-law was the captain of the ship "Empress of Vancouver" on its maiden voyage in the early 1920s, and whose son sailed the Empress on her last voyage, painted an image of the ship to give to his son as a gift.

Nevertheless, a large amount of artwork is created and much of it is put up for public sale. Items displayed in the sales area are in high demand by everyone who visits the center. The residents appreciate the acknowledgment of their work, along with the many positive comments of those who visit the sales exhibit. Artwork Studio sales have also helped to reassure residents' of the value of their artwork, especially those residents who are not able to appreciate the value of their work until someone wants to buy it. Friends that accrue from the public sale of residents' artwork are thus apportioned between the Artworks Program (to cover costs and purchase new materials).

PROGRAM BENEFITS

Becoming a resident of a continuing care facility often occurs after the experience of a great many losses for most people. There are the various perceived losses associated with retirement (e.g., occupation, prestige, power). There are losses related to health and functional ability, including loss of skills developed over a lifetime. Residents also experience a loss of independence, their home, and the life they used to have, as well as the loss of loved ones and friends. Appreciating this context of loss, but also recognizing the continuing potential for growth in later life, the Artworks Studio program contributes to an overall sense of quality of life, purpose, and enjoyment for residents at George Derby Centre. Although they are not able to continue working in their past occupations, homes, or workshops, the Artworks Studio offers residents an opportunity to work with their hands and experience an outlet for creative expression. It does not offer limited, albeit pleasant, activities that serve to help fill the often empty, long hours of an institutional care setting. Rather, the Artworks Studio program provides a means for reengaging "the world of doing, playing, and accomplishing things" (Cath, 2001).

Many of the residents become deeply involved in art-making activities, and experience making art as both an invigorating and calming activity that offers an opportunity for creative self-expression and personal growth, relational connections, and means for affirming the possibilities of later life. Through the process of being involved in art making, residents often experience a heightened sense of well-being. As feelings of anxiety and depression lessen, the residents experience a renewed sense of purpose, self-determination and pride in their work, as well as an enlivened and aesthetically enriched experiencing of the world.

Following Csikszentmihalyi's (1990) theory of flow experiences, the creative art-making experiences that the Artworks Studio program offers can be viewed as helping residents to "develop a stronger, more confident self, because their psychic energy has been invested successfully in goals they themselves had chosen to pursue" (p. 40). "The self becomes more differentiated as a result of flow because overcoming a challenge inevitably leaves a person feeling more capable, more skilled" (p. 41).

In many ways, the instructional ethos underlying the program can be likened to Csikszentmilhalyi's (1990) "flow theory" of optimal experience that outlines conditions associated with experience of "joy, creativity, the process of total involvement with life" (p. xi). Csikszentmihalyi (1990) describes several elements that contribute to flow experiences. He suggests that flow is initiated by focusing one's attention and energy on achieving a challenging, yet realistic, goal-directed activity that requires one's concentrated attention, such that there is a merging of attention and action. This level of involvement in the moment, attending to what one is doing "removes from awareness the worries and frustrations of everyday life" (pp. 59, 61). Often an altered sense of time accompanies the flow experience, and the feeling of the "doing" of the activity itself is the reward. Csikszentmihalyi (1990) suggests that flow experiences can contribute to an overall sense of wholeness and personal meaning, by ". . .integrating one's actions into a unified flow experience that is imbued with a sense of overall purpose" (p. 214). He also claims that expressive activities that attempt to externalize subjective experience (such as storytelling, singing, dance, art, etc.) provide potent conditions for experiencing flow, noting that "in the course of normal life there are few opportunities to experience the feeling of wholeness expressivity provides" (p. 188). He also notes that growth will only occur if it occurs within an enjoyable context that offers "nontrivial opportunities for action and requires a constant perfection of skills" (p. 65).

Through art making, then, the residents become more aware of themselves, others, and the world outside of themselves, and thus become more involved in the world in an intense and alive way. Residents, family members, and staff are reminded about the potency of being alive, of sharing and enjoying creative artworks with one another. The emphasis of the program is not on art making as an individualistic, object-related activity, but on art making as an aesthetic, social, and communicative experience or dialogue; this helps to foster and enrich the development of relationships and a sense of belonging, and also serves to *create* community and culture. Public displays and exhibits of the residents' artwork are an important means of sharing their creative efforts with the larger community. Opportunities for the involvement of family, friends, and elementary and high school students are also an important aspect of the Artworks Studio program. For those residents who become involved in the program and their family members who take an interest, a new activity is found that serves to support an ongoing shared, creative connection. Often, communication can be a challenge, particularly for residents who have lost their speech due to a stroke, and this creative expression becomes an alternative means of communication. Some family members may suggest projects for their relative to make for other family members such as a newborn grandchild or a wedding present. Intergenerational projects offer an opportunity for the residents to share stories, experience, and skills with students who also share stories of their lives.

Stephen Nachmanovich (1990) suggests that the experience of "shared art making is, in and of itself, the expression of, the vehicle for, and the stimulus to human relationships" (p. 99). He suggests that it is through art that we generate and enhance a sense of belonging to a community that we have helped to create. Thus, the Artworks Studio must be viewed not only in terms of its contribution to the wellness of the residents, but the wellness of the community at the George Derby Centre, as well as the larger community of which the centre is a part.

CONCLUSION

This chapter has focused on the power of art making for enlivening one's life, supporting relationships, and fostering community within and beyond the institutional care setting. The Artworks Studio program illustrates a range of possibilities for developing an exemplary arts program in a long-term care setting. Further, it suggests a vision for the arts in long-term care institutions that does not limit "the arts" to time or place, or even a specific purpose, but rather integrates the arts within the everyday life of the institution as "a mode of being," that has resulted in a convergence of "art and life" (Gergen & Gergen, 2001).

We recognize that the George Derby Centre, in part because of government funding from Veteran's Affairs Canada and concern for honoring veterans for their war efforts, offers a superior complement of arts programming that may be difficult to emulate in other settings. Nevertheless, our hope is that all of those involved in creating residential communities for seniors (policymakers, program planners, professional health care teams, and seniors themselves) will recognize the creative capacity of older adults. The potential of lifelong learning and growth in later life is vast, and the benefits of the arts for all of those living and working within a continuing care community are far-reaching. We hope that other residential communities will learn from this, and work to incorporate comprehensive arts programming as an integral component of these communities.

REFERENCES

Alexander, T. M. (1987). *John Dewey's theory of art, experience, and nature.* Albany, NY: State University of New York Press.

Canadian Red Cross Society. (1989). *An instructors guide to crafts for special needs.* Vancouver, BC: The Canadian Red Cross Society, Arts and Crafts Department, BC/ Yukon Division.

Cath, S. H. (2001). Foreward: Empathic connections. In N. Weisburg & R. Wilder (Eds.), *Expressive arts with elders: A resource.* London: Jessica Kingsley.

Csikszentmihalyi, M. (1990). *Flow: The psychology of optimal experience.* New York: Harper & Row.

Dewey, J. (1934). *Art as experience.* New York: Minton, Balch & Co.

Dissanayake, E. (1992). *Homo aestheticus: Where art comes from and why.* New York: Free Press.

Eisner, E. W. (1972). *Educating artistic vision.* New York: Macmillan.

Gergen, K. J., & Gergen, M. (2001). *Aging as creative reconstruction.* Paper presented at the meeting of the International Association on Gerontology, 17th World Congress, Vancouver, BC (Canada).

Hoffman, D. H. (1992). *Arts for older adults: An enhancement of life.* Englewood Cliffs, NJ: Prentice Hall.

Hubalek, S. K. (1998). Training personnel to teach art to older adults living in special care facilities. In D. H, Fitzner & M. M. Rugh (Eds.), *Crossroads: The challenge of lifelong learning.* Reston, VI: The National Art Education Association.

London, P. (1989). *No more second hand art: Awakening the artist within.* Boston: Shambahla.

Nachmanovich, S. (1990). *Free play: The power of improvisation in life and the arts.* Los Angeles, CA: Jeremy P. Tarcher.

Stokrocki, M. L. (1998). A participant observation study of an art class for physically-challenged adults. In D. H, Fitzner & M. M. Rugh (Eds.), *Crossroads: The challenge of lifelong learning.* Reston, VI: The National Art Education Association.

Weisburg, N., & Wilder, R. (Eds.). (2001). *Expressive arts with elders: A resource.* London: Jessica Kingsley.

SECTION II

WORKING WITH SPECIFIC
OLDER ADULT POPULATIONS

Chapter 5

MEETING YOUR METAPHOR: THE USE OF THE ARTS AND THE IMAGINATION WITH DYING PERSONS

Denis Whalen

WORKING WITH METAPHORS

A metaphor can be a way of naming something that feels too big, frightening, and/or overwhelming to talk about in everyday language. By definition, a metaphor is a figure of speech, often found in poetry, that describes one thing in terms of another; for example, "the evening of life" to describe the later years of life. It is a way to be more precise and accurate in naming our thoughts and feelings instead of accepting the general definition, which is usually a label. An accurate personal naming of something gives us a better chance of easing into something universal and can help us stand outside of our experience and ourselves.

A personal, "just right" metaphor can be particularly helpful in finding a healthy distance from the existential anxiety around dying, a way to be with the unknown. In many ways, the unknown is the essence of the artistic process itself. If we can invite that metaphor in for a cup of tea, we have a better chance of finding a way to hold the strong feelings we have around the experience. Some of the normal and persistent feelings that dying persons have include: fear, anger, frustration, hopelessness, helplessness, sadness, and grief. How can metaphor help the dying person move these thoughts and feelings around, so that they can be given tender attention, aired out, irrigated, and, perhaps, reframed as resources and strengths?

I believe that the arts can be helpful as tools in organizing and shaping the most precise and poetic metaphor for the shifting and evolving moments of a person's life.

Although the metaphor is important in and of itself, even more essential is the skillful dexterity of meeting and mapping the metaphor as thoughts and feelings shift and evolve over the course of a day, an illness, a lifetime. A metaphor that fits one day for one moment or one person can move like the tide, ebbing and flowing with our thoughts and emotions. It is my feeling that metaphors need updating on a regular basis.

In my work as coordinator of a center which serves those diagnosed with Amyotrophic Lateral Sclerosis, more commonly known as Lou Gehrig's disease or ALS, I have used the language of the arts, writing, drawing, music, and dancing to facilitate finding one's own metaphor in meeting the challenges of this condition. ALS is a progressive neuromuscular condition that affects all of the voluntary muscles, resulting in weakness and paralysis. In addition to affecting the physical functions of mobility, eating, speaking, and breathing with death usually coming within two to five years of diagnosis, the psychological and emotional challenges of this condition are often overwhelming, not only to the patient but also to the caregivers. Cognitively intact, patients often feel like they are trapped in a body that has failed them. They understandably feel anger at what has interrupted their life and dreams. Frustration runs high around not being able to communicate easily when the facial muscles become too weak to produce speech. Even with the sophisticated technology of adapted computers, communication can become laborious. Understandably, they experience fears of being a burden to family and caregivers, of helplessness, and ultimately of dying. Time after time, my experience has shown me how the arts can give the patient and caregivers a way to respond to their suffering. I have used the original artwork of the patient, the artwork created by the caregiver as a response to the patient, and the rich and diverse material from already created art. In this chapter, I will share a few stories about some remarkable people who embraced their metaphors as they lived their dying.

Sometimes a person comes upon a metaphor on his/her own, as Norm did. A painter and sculptor all his life, he created a sculpture when he was diagnosed with ALS. He directed a group of his artist friends to cut down a living apple tree from his backyard, strip off the bark, and lay it down on the floor of his studio. This recumbent shape was decorated with plaster models of motor neurons that were breaking apart. He and his family, along with all his fellow artists, mourned their collective losses in the making and exhibition of this artwork.

However, many times people need some tools to help them discover a personal metaphor for the reality of being diagnosed with a terminal illness. From my experience, dying persons often express a desire to leave a legacy, engage in a reevaluative life review process in order to make peace with their life, mourn their losses, and find a way to say goodbye to their loved ones. Using a combination of art-based modalities is a powerful way to meet these needs, allowing a person to access resources and creativity to shape their own solutions. *The expressive arts therapy* approach to using the arts is a nonthreatening process that requires no artistic training, only a willingness to explore one's own inner territory. Daria Halprin (2003), in her book, *The Expressive Body in Life, Art and Therapy*, says, "The way we work with the creative process and the arts is very different from that of the artist who immerses herself in art for art's sake, or who shapes her art in order to deliver a message to her audience. We work with the arts metaphorically, as a way of identifying, reflecting on, and changing our conditioning. We work with art and the creative process as a paradigm for addressing suffering" (p. 19).

CASE STUDIES

Amber: Riding the Waves

I visited Amber at her home once a week for almost a year. A single parent with three children, she had been diagnosed with ALS one year earlier. Early in our work together, she chose an image of a spider's web. She played with this image, expanding its significance from trap, to safety net, to Internet, seeing the multiple meanings in a single image. She seemed to know that by seeing various meanings, she had a better chance of seeing the multifaceted nature of her own situation, reminding me of the Cubist perspective of "holding multiple perspectives simultaneously." Saki Santorelli (1999) in his book, *Heal Thy Self*, defines healing as ". . . our willingness to feel and hold all parts of ourselves in awareness without division and distinction" (p. 130). Out of a dialogue with this and other images, Amber created a number of poems that were assembled into a book to be given to her children. [Note: The poems and writings that appear in this book are published by permission of their authors or the families of the authors.]

The Swing

When I was small
the world seemed so large.
I remember swinging on my swing,
Higher and higher I would go
up above the trees like a bird.
I would look down on the rooftops.
I felt invincible.
The wind would blow in my face on the way down.
My hair would blow in the wind on the my way up.
As an adult, my world has become quite small.
I no longer have the feelings of a child
or feel the freedom of the wind against my face.
There are certain feelings
that we can only experience once.
For me it's that old swing.

Untitled

I saw this picture of a bike.
It was parked on a dock in
the middle of a lake.
I couldn't help but wonder how it got there.
There were no boats or people near it.
It seemed so out of place.
I realized at that moment that
that is how I feel about ALS.
It's here, it's a reality
but I don't know how it got here
and it seems so out of place.
It doesn't fit into my life.
It doesn't fit in my children's life.
But yet it's here, like that
bike, waiting for someone or
something to come and take it away.

He Is Near

When all is quiet
and darkness has filled the room,
I come to the Lord in prayer.
He whispers back and lets me know He's near.
I tell Him about my day.
He tells me He already knows.
He was there when I cried
and didn't know why.
He gave me peace.
He was there when I lashed
out in anger.
He gave me understanding.
He was there when I felt weak.
He gave me strength.
He was there when I felt all alone.
He gave me comfort.
As the light of a new day fills the room,
He gives the best gift of all,
His unconditional love.

Sunflowers

I've always had a love of sunflowers,
their majestic beauty,
the way they seem to be
looking over the garden
with their golden petals beaming. . .
almost the way a mother
looks at her child.

To our sessions, I often brought a bag of different textured items and asked Amber to choose something from the bag with her eyes closed that described how she was feeling at that particular moment, a sort of emotional temperature game. Below are a few of the things that she chose and what she said about them.

"I am a tangled hunk of yarn with some feathers intertwined," she said. She continues to talk about the softness of the yarn, and how it reminded her of a body losing tone and neurons, a body off-key that feels soft and yielding and not up to doing the simplest things. I silently asked myself, "How is it to live inside this softness, inside a body that can't do the simplest things?" One day she chose a rock and said,

"I am a flat, oblong stone, washed smooth by the ocean." And then added, "People don't realize how impaired I am. They think I should be able to do the same things I could do a few weeks ago and I can't. And I can't make myself understood . . . I run into a stone wall."

When she picked out something rumpled and metallic, she said, "I am a crumpled piece of aluminum foil. I am folding into myself like an accordion. I can't move around in bed. I get stuck." On this occasion, I understand this feeling of being stuck in my own life, and Amber's naming of this phenomenon ignites a sense of kinship with her.

Sometimes this exercise of naming and questioning led to practical problem solving with the occupational therapist on the homecare team. More often, it became an opportunity for both of us to see the enormity of the losses being endured and also the strength of the human spirit to find a way to live as fully as possible with whatever was happening in life at any one moment. Amber began to come into an appreciative awareness of her resources, and our relationship deepened into a collaborative exchange between two human beings. Although many team members had questioned Amber's understanding of the seriousness of her situation (because of her perceived reluctance to make practical plans for her own care and that of her children), sharing Amber's words with them helped to give them a sense of her deep personal suffering and her understanding of her reality.

As she approached the last stages of her illness, Amber began to make decisions about the use of extraordinary measures at the end of life, choosing a health care proxy and guardians for her youngest children. The image of relentless waves and a resilient surfer came up a number of times and I wrote a poem for her as an aesthetic response to her awesome ability to stay engaged in her world in the face of her increasing disability. She was touched by this gesture and began to allow a deeper level of trust and intimacy with me and others around her. She acknowledged the need for more family members, friends, and volunteers to become involved not only with her care but also with her children's.

Wave-walker
Rogue-surfer

Sometimes the tidal wave
Sometimes the puny surfer

Finding your balance
Perched on the edge

A glorious glide into the shore
or a wild crashing into the sea
Either way
Only those who have been in the ocean
know you can't stop the waves
They are the ones who learn how to surf

Amber took to poetry and metaphor like a duck to water. She used her lively imagination to accurately name her feelings, which brought her into greater awareness of what was happening in her life. Just this simple act of accurately and precisely naming what was in front of her eyes was enough to help her stay with important questions such as the practical day-to-day issues around her own care and her children's—the difficult decision to agree to Hospice care and the existential questions around her own dying and leaving her young children. The arts did not give her the answers. It gave her tools to become aware of her own deep resources of compassion and common sense.

Margot: Angel's Wings

Margot, an older woman diagnosed with ALS, was referred to me by another staff member. My co-worker thought that working with images would be a way to externalize and give form to the thoughts and feelings that Margot seemed to be having difficulty putting into words. When I first met Margot, she communicated by writing, having lost the ability to speak a few months earlier. After a brief introduction about what our work together might be, Margot wrote "Art . . . I'm not good at that." This is a common response, especially from older adults, who often consider art making as reserved for a special class of "artists" and not available to them in their everyday life. This is the place where I find the theory of Expressive Arts Therapy can be helpful in reassuring a person that creating and shaping art is something we do naturally everyday of our lives. Just the simple act of choosing our clothing is a creative act that most of us do every day. We talked about creating art with "low skill and high sensitivity," one of the foundational concepts of expressive arts. It is also helpful to point out that the value of making art is in the act of making, not in the finished product. It is the process of shaping a metaphor, how the person is in this process, and how he/she perceives it that can be most helpful.

Working Through Resistance

I have often heard Director and Founder of Glass Lake Studio, Geoffrey Scott-Alexander say that "How you are in painting (or any kind of art making) is how you are in life." For instance, do we stay with the work even when it becomes difficult? How strong is the critic inside of us and how willing are we to step out of our own way to allow something to emerge naturally? Noticing these things can come out of participation in the art-making process and can point to our resources. The other aspect of art making that can sometimes be a stumbling block is the perception of art and art making as useless or self-indulgent activity, tangential to real life, and unproductive. Often I hear a critical statement that "this is child's play" and not worthwhile or appropriate for grown-ups. A lighthearted approach works best here, pointing out that creating art is "high play," a very relaxed, playful approach with a very serious intention. I also suggest to the person that we work with already created art, such as reading his/her favorite poetry, listening to music, and looking at familiar visual art and creating collages from photos and magazine images. This way the focus shifts to the process, to their response and away from the making of a "beautiful" finished product.

During our first session together, Margot chose some images from the National Geographic magazines that I brought with me: a man standing under a rocky cave, many nature scenes, pairs of animals that made her laugh as she identified them as "Margot and Ron," she and (I), and an ocean scene which prompted me to put ocean music on the CD player. Then she began to choose some words from the "word bowl," a collection of words and phrases cut from magazines and newspapers, and glued them on some of the images. She was attracted to an image of trees and branches, bare of leaves, surrounded by fog and standing in water, maybe a swamp. She was able to verbally finish the sentence that I started, *I am finding myself*. . ."feeling blue." Then she picked up a blue oil pastel and covered a piece of paper with sinuous blue lines. For someone who proclaims herself to be "not good at art," she jumped right in and did a lot of work during the first session.

When I returned a few weeks later, some other images that she had chosen the last time had been glued down on a large piece of paper. She pointed to the empty spaces and proceeded to choose more images. She then wrote a few words about a photo of three chairs overlooking a lake, "a beautiful place where I can have some peace." A photo of two elderly ladies reminded her of her grandmother and she imagined a conversation between them and wrote it down. Margot confirmed my belief in everyone's natural ability to enliven the images and go right into them, speak with them, and listen as they talk back. She returned to the image that attracted her so strongly the last time, the trees standing in the water and I suggested that she write a poem inspired by this image. I guided her through a poetic structure called diamante, which is created from seven lines using a sequence of nouns, adjectives, and verbs. I find that this structure puts a secure frame around the process.

> Foreboding
> shadowy, nothing
> drowning, drying, weeping
> loneliness, darkness, angel's wings
> fly, away, escape
> lonely, dark
> tree-world

The "angel's wings" came from Margot's transposing of letters in the word, "angles;" this was a surprise and she decided to leave it in. Margot did not appear to be distressed by these images. Her husband, who never actively participated in a session but was always within earshot while Margot and I worked, looked over her shoulder and mentioned that he had dark thoughts sometimes too. Margot accepted this collage as a "self-portrait" for the day, a container for some her thoughts and feelings, normal and understandable, and so often left unsaid. Collage can be a more truthful way of telling a complex life story because it captures the way life is lived—not with a linear story line, but with things happening in the piecemeal and overlapping way that we all know to be the way it is. After this session, I sent Margot an acrostic poem built on the letters of her name.

> like eMbers
> on the heArth
> remembeRing
> secret sonGs
> Of
> Tenderness

I only had the privilege of working with Margot a couple of times. Although personally she enjoyed and felt comfortable with the arts and expression, there were strong cultural pressures to remain stoic and quiet. However, her daughter became a regular at the caregivers' group at the center and it seemed to me that the effect of the work was more easily seen in her ability to share her grief with others in the group. Additionally, through the expressive work we did in the group, she found a way to access her reservoirs of compassion for herself as she cared for her mother and provided support for her father.

Rita: "Phenomenal Phlamingo"

Rita and I worked together as patient and Occupational Therapist, as willing guinea pig and Expressive Art Therapist-in-training, and finally as companions on our life journeys for over a year. During that time, Rita moved from a leadership position in state government to someone who could not move any voluntary muscles, including those of speech and swallowing. There were many practical and important adaptation issues that my OT background could help to solve. However, neither one of us lost sight of the essential work of doing an artful life review, communicating and expressing her thoughts and feelings, and leaving a legacy to her husband and two grown children.

My professor, Geoffrey Scott-Alexander, Registered Expressive Arts Therapist and Founder/Director of the Glass Lake Studio in Albany, New York, facilitated one of the first groups that Rita attended. All of the participants were asked to identify an animal that they felt attracted to or had a special interest in. Geoffrey helped each person to expand the animal into a metaphor that had something to say about his/her individual resources and strengths. Rita chose a unique power animal, a flamingo. She liked how flamingos could stand in the mud and yet at the same time be high above everything, an image for her of being immersed in the "mud" of ALS, yet able to have a healthy distance, a longer view that helped put things into perspective. She maintained this "flamingo essence" until her death and I think it accounted for her ability live in the opposites; for example, to hold the qualities of intimacy and remoteness simultaneously, which allowed her to live with a touching dignity.

I tried nearly everything with Rita and she was open to experimentation. We made life collages. I acted out some of the humorous stories from her childhood. I literally stood on my head when everything else failed. She did not "like" poetry but I kept trying. However we never found anything that felt like synchronous expression for her. She did like what I referred to, tongue-in-cheek, as "trashy" novels and we read them together. Her son, Scott, was one of her primary caregivers, a skilled musician and music major at a nearby college. Rita loved to hear him talk about the music he loved, and during the school year when he was away, we would listen to the music we knew he was practicing and performing at school. During this time, I was assembling a loose-leaf notebook of meditation images, photographs, and drawings of different things (flowers, animals, scenes from nature, an old pair of shoes, a doorway), and poetry that accompanied the images. I would offer this book as a resource to individuals and if something attracted them, an image or poem they would like to work with, I would just remove it from the binder and give it to them to keep. Rita and I watched videos together, read a play together, cooked together, anything that could help us fall in love with something larger than ourselves, to care about something outside of ourselves and that nurtured a trusting relationship with each other. I drew pictures of flamingos and wrote "once upon a time" stories about them. Her family was amazed when Rita wrote a poem based on the title of her life review journal, "Rita Remembering."

fRiends
forEver
Make
lifE
Merry
Because
Each day
Reminds
me sIlently
of the preseNce
of God

One day, Rita announced that she wanted to write letters to her children on her adapted computer. She used an on-screen keyboard and a special switch and letter by letter, Rita painstakingly wrote letters filled with reminiscences and farewell wishes. For her birthday, a few months before she died, I adapted the poem "Phenomenal

Woman" by Maya Angelou into "Phenomenal Phlamingo." A small plush pink flamingo still sits on my computer as a reminder of our relationship.

Countertransference

I think it is only natural that at some point during such intimate work as this, a patient or client comes along who resonates deeply with your own essence, your values, beliefs, and feelings. As I look back from my perspective today, I see that Rita and I shared some similar life experiences and that I was deeply touched by her and what was happening to her. I became more involved with her and her family than I ever had before. Because there were no family members living in the area, I volunteered to organize the neighbors and friends into a care team and became one of the team members, spending every Thursday afternoon with Rita. When the time came for the committal service of Rita's ashes, a year and a half after her death, her husband asked me to write a few words about Rita that could be read at the service.

This experience became an opportunity for me to know deep down, the power of the arts for myself as a professional caregiver. I realized how important it is to do our own work, every day. I was lucky to be involved in my expressive arts training program through this period and found many ways to use the arts to stay with my own questions about disability, helplessness, the frustration of running out of "fix-it" answers, and finally understanding how to really just be there *with* someone, not there *for* them. An experience of dramatic enactment helped me to see my relationships from another perspective and how the lines of communication, actually strung out between the characters with colored crepe paper, were becoming entwined. It was a powerful learning for me, an in-the-body-learning, experience that didn't give me an answer as much as it gave me new eyes for seeing reality and the possibilities within it.

The metaphor that reminds me of my relationship with Rita is the Zen rock garden, a hard place of extraordinary beauty and tension. I see three or four uniquely shaped rocks on a bed of sand. The rocks are still and the sand is raked into patterns around them. The pattern tends to become fuzzy and needs to be reestablished every time we meet. Sometimes I'm the rocks and Rita is the sand and sometimes we reverse roles. Rocks and sand in relation to one another guide us to see things in a new way—reality and unreality in a dance. Like all gardens, this one operates on natural time, which requires slowing down. In this garden, I confronted my preconceptions of what life should be. What I found in there was something so radically different it called forth a deeper response, empty of clutter; this allowed me to see the world in a new way, to see the cosmic in, every day and to see the whole world in a grain of sand.

> To see a World in a Grain of Sand
> And a Heaven in a Wild Flower,
> Hold Infinity in the palm of your hand
> And Eternity in an hour.
> -William Blake

Rita's use of metaphor was complex and in some ways became the connector between everyone involved in her care: the neighbors, the professionals, and the family members. The original metaphor, discovered very early in her illness, the flamingo, became a window into Rita's "way" that she was choosing to follow. A way that was both realistic, as seen in her early decision to have a feeding tube before her swallowing difficulties became severe and her acceptance of adaptive equipment and technology, and at the same time imaginative, with a touch of riding above the mud on the long legs of the fairy tale.

Arlene: The Niverville Rascal

Arlene was a hearty woman who had great physical strength all her life, a gritty perspective on life, and a robust sense of humor grounded in nature and the simple things of life. Her highest values were centered on helping her family and friends. (This nickname, the Niverville Rascal, comes from the name of her hometown and the brand name of the scooter she used to get around in the neighborhood.) She had written poetry for years, a way of celebrating the special events in the lives of her loved ones. When she was diagnosed with ALS, it was only natural that Arlene would go to poetry, first as a way to communicate with her caregivers and, once in a while, to express some of her fears. For instance, she was embarrassed and baffled by her uncontrollable crying. "I swear I won't do this and it happens," she said. (ALS can sometimes affect a part of the brain that monitors emotional responses, resulting in so-called "inappropriate" or labile crying and laughing.) It is helpful to understand some of the physiological rationales behind behavior. However, given Arlene's situation of being diagnosed with a progressive and terminal condition, emotional expression becomes understandable and necessary. Arlene said that she never cried much during her life, so this was an unfamiliar place to be. She began to feel like she did not know who she any more. Her "job" of taking care of other people was slowly being taken away as her muscles became weaker and she was unable to move around. I would hear her say, "I can't do anything." Her speech was severely affected and she began to communicate exclusively by writing. Her handwriting was still graceful and flowing. While working on a collage together, Arlene chose a computer-generated image of a spider spinning her web. In the image, the progression of the process was shown by using different colors to show which strands were laid down first, then next etc.; from this image came words like puzzle, webbing, spider, stringing, weaving, threading. A poem came . . . to be finished later. Arlene began to cry too hard to continue our work together, so we spent the next half hour just sitting together. This was a work in progress and I hoped to continue working with Arlene and encouraging her to use her gift of poetical expression to explore this time of her life and come to some awareness of her beauty and strengths, and perhaps understanding and meaning of what was happening in her life.

As the disease progressed, Arlene began sending her poems to other members of the ALS team: her doctor, who responded with a poem of his own, the Speech Therapist, and the Occupational Therapy students who interned at the center. Her 12-year-old grandson began writing poetry to her, and assembled together a book of his poems for her. Somehow poetry writing itself became the metaphor for Arlene; even when coherent speech was not longer possible and she could no longer type or hold the pen, she was always the poet laureate of the ALS Center.

Linda: Living in the Layers

In addition to my work with persons with ALS, I facilitate art experiences with dying persons through a unique program of complementary therapies offered by the community hospice received in our area. I had a call to visit Linda, a cancer patient, and was asked to call her as soon as possible to set up a visit because it was believed she was very near death. Due to her pain medication, she was not able to work very long and drifted in and out of attention during the hour we spent together. She showed me her art journal and pages of meticulous, multicolored mosaic paintings/drawings. The colors were jewel bright and each geometric of color was precisely outlined with black and stacked on the page in layers. I suggested she have a dialog with one of her drawings and ask it if it had anything to tell her. She warmed to this idea because she had already made several spontaneous comments about the aliveness of the images for her, so it was just a small leap into personifying the images and listening to them speak. A list of words was generated: "blossoming," "organizing," "systematizing," "loving," "sleeping." Linda then began to build a poem using some of these words. She looked back and forth between the drawings and the poem, saying how she saw her life now, "one layer at a time," how she had built it up in layers, like the colored shapes in her drawing, and that she saw her children building in the same way. I am reminded of a poem by Stanley Kunitz called "The Layers" and shared the few lines with her that I remembered.

When I look behind,
as I am compelled to look
before I can gather strength
to proceed on my journey,
I see the milestones dwindling
toward the horizon . . .
(and then further on in the poem):
. . . Live in the layers,
not on the litter (p. 107).

She fussed and rearranged the words, then smiled, as she saw the meticulous attention to order in her drawings and how she was working with her words . . . just a little gentle acceptance for how it was, how she was. This is a good example of the nonjudgmental attitude that is at the heart of expressive arts therapy, not only toward the artwork being created but also towards ourselves. At this point, I introduced a collection of meditation images and poetry that I had assembled and she said she would like to put a similar book together using her original drawings and poetry. Linda was inspired to leave a message for her young children as the symmetry of her drawings reflected the layers of her experience and how she had nurtured her children within those layers; this helped her to come to some peace about their being able to go on with their lives. As she explored the creation story of her artwork she wrote a long poem, which she shared with her mother that afternoon. I received a call from the social worker the next day that Linda had died the next morning.

Linda had done her work before I walked in the door. She had all of the pieces, the layers if you will, like a patchwork quilt ready to be sewn together. All she needed was a frame. By holding the space for her to be with her layered images, a poem naturally emerged from them. The poems, like her children, were nurtured within and came directly out of those layers.

EXPRESSIVE ARTS THERAPY IN-SERVICES

Some of my work involves giving in-services to Hospice board members, administrators, staff members, and volunteers, as well as teaching classes in the bereavement program at an area college on using the arts with dying persons. I begin with the necessity of looking at our own mortality and how we are with our own losses and grief. I ask them to listen to the stories of others and how they faced their dying, how using the arts and artful living helped them, and to imagine how it might help us someday.

In the experiential component of these workshops and presentations, I ask the participants to give form to the thoughts and feelings that emerge from hearing the stories, perhaps using oil pastels on paper, closing their eyes, and using their nondominant hand to short circuit one's inner critic. Then perhaps some words come from the drawing that may flow into a poem or a phrase. Even one word can be a gift. Using the arts in combination allows a range of modalities for just the right fit between what wants to be expressed, and the style and preferences of the person. The experience can be deepened by going into gesture or movement if time and inclination allows.

IDEAS FOR PRACTICE

Here are some exercises to try in the nonjudgmental spirit of expressive arts therapy. It is important to stay attuned to the physical and emotional energy of the person you are working with. Sometimes just listening and responding to a piece of music will be the work and other times the person may be able to engage more actively in the creative process by writing a poem or creating a piece of art.

1. Help your client explore the opposites found in nature and in human experience; begin by talking about the range of emotions and responses that are possible. For example, sometimes we are the tidal wave (the one who is powerful), sometimes the puny surfer (the one who is struggling); sometimes we say yes and sometimes no. We are capable of responding to our life from anywhere along this continuum and we can make our choices from this wide range if we become aware of it.

   The next step in this process is to choose images from a magazine, (*National Geographic* is a good source), that say something about the range of a quality or situation that the client has chosen to work with today, perhaps their own sense of helplessness and their own sense of capability, their own way of saying yes and their own way of saying no. Then create a collage out of the images, either gluing them onto a large piece of paper or connecting them one to the other but not gluing them down. Then the collage can act as an oracle, answering questions, speaking directly to the person. If personifying the work of art is difficult, then a discussion can be had about the process of making the collage, how the images are arranged, what was easy or difficult about the process and what were the surprises. Possibly discuss where the images merge and diverge. Think about the fact that if they can live together on the page, perhaps they can live together within a person and his/her life situation.

2. Have your client choose a quality like power, love, compassion, or anger, and write down as many words as possible that he/she associates with this quality. For instance, if you were working with "power," you might have "water, money, red, the Madonna, shark, tree" etc. Make a long list, using colors, historical figures,

poems, animals, whatever. Let your imagination roam. Look over the list and choose two words or phrases that feel like they say something about the continuum of "power" from gentle to strong, perhaps the Madonna and the shark. You can now work with these images in a number of ways. Try starting out by writing a sentence claiming the distinct power of these images for yourself. "I have the compassionate heart of the Madonna that can hold the sorrow of the world." And, "Beware of my toothy grin as I cut through the water looking for a meal." The question then becomes can he/she claim the power at either end of this continuum?

3. Suggest enjoying already created art by going to a museum for an hour or two, reading some poetry by Emily Dickinson, Walt Whitman, W.B. Yeats, or any poet of your choice, or listening to some beautiful music. Plant some seeds. Contemplate a flower to experience the beauty of nature. Encourage your client to notice that there is something beautiful in him/her that resonates within him/her when you appreciate beauty in nature and in the masterpieces of art.

4. Here is something to try in a group or family setting. Working in dyads, have the group members tell a two-minute story to the other person about someone (other than a family member) who has had a big influence on his/her life. Take turns listening and telling stories among the pair. After this you have material to work with, choose images and materials to create a collage out of this story. Let the images choose you. Our stories are more like collage than a line drawing, with things popping out here and there, not in a linear way, one thing following another in a predictable and orderly fashion. See if there are any surprises in the images the group members choose. Have the members share their collage with one another, or, if you are working in a larger group, perhaps with the whole group.

5. Begin with a centering exercise, bringing attention to the breathing and guiding your client through a body scan. Have the person remain in a comfortable position and suggest that they begin rolling a short movie in his/her head of the events of his/her life during the last week, last year, or whatever time frame you would like to work with. After ten or fifteen minutes, have the client come back to the room, and let one scene come to mind, one that

he/she wished had been different; take a pencil and paper and rewrite the scene. He/she is the director, the editor, the rewrite person, and here is his/her chance to make it come out different-ly. Use dialogue and as much detail as possible. Share with a part-ner, or if working individually, with you as therapist. Continue to expand this story by writing a poem or doing some drawing with oil pastels.

6. Suggest that your client try writing a letter to him/herself, to the person he/she is today, from the person he/she was several years ago or vice versa.

7. Using oil pastels, have your client create a series of three abstract drawings, each taking approximately five minutes; the first one will say something about where he/she is now, the second about where he/she wants to be, and the third about what it will take to get there. After the drawings have been done, move the client into writing a "once upon a time" story based on the drawings.

8. Enlarge the available living space, what expressive artists call "play space" by exploring some art modalities that are unfamiliar, such as clay. Have the client knead and manipulate the clay with eyes closed. Explain that there is no need to make it into a rec-ognizable shape, just stay with it for a few minutes and see what happens. Be curious about what happens when you stop trying. Buy a set of watercolors and play with the colors, letting them flow together. Try using musical instruments to "play" the colors. Read Pablo Neruda's poem, "Ode to Common Things" to see with new eyes the everyday objects of our lives. Write an ode, a hymn of praise, to your shoe or the telephone, or the first things you see when you wake up in the morning. Wake up to the beau-ty that is all around us.

MEMORIES AND FINAL WORDS

The following vignettes are snippets of memories of a variety of clients who have touched me. I hope that these stories move you to use the arts to deepen your connection to your own creativity and spir-ituality. Artists have always known that each of us is so much bigger and more beautiful than we ever take the time to imagine. I remember Laurie, whose doctor came to visit her a few days before her death and danced for her, a concert of ballroom dances to celebrate a life well lived. And Marjorie, who directed the making of a dream catcher, personalized by different colored beads that she used to name her fears of dying.

And Bruce, who went to his farm fields in his power wheelchair and when the caregivers left, silently called his beloved dairy cows to his side where they nuzzled and licked him. And Bob, who found his whole world while looking out the window of his living room.

And Fred, who adopted the eagle as his power animal and helper and scanned it onto his computer as a screen saver, where he saw it every day. And Corinne, who shaped a work of ceiling art out of mementos and messages from friends. And Don's family who got out all of the photo albums and as he lay dying, laughed and cried as they wrapped themselves in the beautiful interweavings of their lives together.

And Sharon, who poured the story of her life into the "heirlooms" in her home . . . the carpets, a locket, courting letters, diaries. The use of treasured objects to weave a life story acknowledges the importance of what happens between people and things. Occupational Therapy, a therapy that I believe partners well with Expressive Arts Therapy, uses an "Object History" to raise awareness of the significant linkages between the nonhuman objects of special meaning and a person's life history. This whole area is a rich area to be explored by the imagination and creative arts. Somehow Sharon instinctively knew that giving voice to the objects of her life would be a complete and satisfying way to tell her story.

And Barney, with only the steady rhythm of his ventilator as a sign of his presence in the room as his caregivers of ten years told stories to the videotape machine. John, his 10- year-old son, talked about their shared love of the Jets football team. His home care doctor talked of the triumphs and the difficulties of providing care at home during these years. I remember his wife sitting quietly in the corner, not wanting to be on camera and listening intently. His 24-hour round-the-clock nurses all were present for this celebration of saying goodbye, creating a permanent record for the family.

May the arts bring into your life the tools you and your clients need to embrace stillness and to tell your stories so that they may live. As Thoreau (2000) invites:

It is something to be able to paint a picture, or to carve a statue, and so to make a few objects beautiful. But it is far more glorious to carve and paint the atmosphere in which we work, to effect the quality in which we work, to effect the quality of the day–this is the highest of the arts. (p. 101)

REFERENCES

Halprin, D. (2003). *The expressive body in life, art and therapy.* Philadelphia: Jessica Kingsley Publishers Ltd.

Kunitz, S. (1997). *Passing through: The later poems.* New York: W.W. Norton & Co.

Santorelli, S. (1999). *Heal thy self.* New York: Bell Tower.

Thoreau, H.D. (2000). *Walden and civil disobedience.* New York: Houghton Mifflin Co.

Chapter 6

HOME-BASED ART THERAPY FOR OLDER ADULTS

SHINYA SEZAKI AND JOAN BLOOMGARDEN

INTRODUCTION

The purpose of this paper is to report theoretical background and case studies on art therapy for the elderly living at home. While concrete services such as occupational therapy, physical therapy, and nursing care are usual, psychological services provided at home are rare. Art therapy is versatile; it can be an included service and contribute to satisfying life experiences for the person served as well as his or her significant others. Although the territory of home-based art therapy for elderly homebound adults has not been fully explored, some therapists have broken new ground by providing clinical material and theory on this topic.

Bell (1998) wrote about his experiences of home-based therapy as a hospice worker in the United Kingdom. Gibson (1994) wrote about the home-based elderly, and called for home intervention to avoid the homebound elderly from equating "old = illness = death." She notes how the art therapist can assist a person to retrieve independence through art making, giving the elder patient an opportunity to gain self-esteem. Lindblad-Goldberg, Dore & Stern (1998) wrote a comprehensive text on the general structure of home-based family services and the challenges faced in clinical work and supervision. Although they are not art therapists, their focused knowledge of family systems, social work, and program development all relate to the art therapy clinician planning to work in the home setting.

These resources assisted the first author's care and treatment plan for three homebound elderly adults. The following presents a general discussion of home-based art therapy and the role of the art therapist as seen by the co-authors during a one-year clinical experience in domiciliary services.

HOME-BASED ART THERAPY

Within the field of art therapy Gibson (1994), with her understanding of gerontology, argues that art therapy can provide a unique home-based mental health service to confront various mental distresses, including serious depression. Bell (1998) discusses home-based art therapy in palliative care in the United Kingdom. He claims that for terminally ill people who are taken care of in their home, psychological care and support become crucial, especially when they have a problem in communicating with their caregivers or other family members at an emotional level. Based on his practice as an art therapist in a hospice, Bell (1998) supports art therapy in the home and says:

> Despite the puzzlement that often greets me on my first visit to the family home, art therapy is a very accessible means for people to communicate their profound emotional needs. The lack of familiarity with art therapy is soon overcome once the patient has experimented with the process of creating an image and grasps the connection between the content of the picture and their interests, memories, ideas, opinions, experiences of ill health and the implications for them of a life-threatening disease. (p. 100)

Much of traditional art therapy training can be applied to home-based treatment; however, this special environment has its own set of needs and a unique structure that calls for distinctive and individual approaches to art therapy. Just as the therapist must understand the differences between individual therapy and group therapy, the in-home therapist needs to understand the differences between institutional and home-based practice. Basically, home-based therapists must learn new roles, techniques, and obligations when they start to work with clients and their families in this specialized setting. Lindblad-Goldberg, et al. (1998) explain that "home-based practice potentially exposes the therapist to the seven "C's": chaos, crisis, cross-system complexity, cultural sensitivity, collaboration, competence, and change" (p. 24). To help navigate a complex multiproblem situation, they describe ways to work with the families' own internal resources.

Home-based work can draw on all available strengths both from the community and from supportive caregivers who offer possibilities to learn and be creative. It is generally agreed that the home is the least restrictive setting of all sites where the elderly live, allowing for diversity of treatments and ideas. The perception of the elderly as being problematic individuals to people who can engage in purposeful activities requires a paradigm shift "from the fountain of youth to the fountain of age" (Kerr, 1999, p. 40).

It is widely argued in gerontology that many older patients lose their independence and become depressed in an institutional setting (Atchley, 1987); and when asked, most of older patients prefer home-based care (Melcher, 1988). For a therapist, the home provides valuable information about his or her clients and their support group. By observing the clients' belongings, their room, and their interaction with the family, the therapist becomes familiar with the clients' individual history, culture, and information that helps create a holistic treatment approach. Knowing which family members can be involved and when strengthens the possibilities and lessens false expectations and stresses. While institutional care can also provide creative activities, the larger dimension of the home offers broader choices and additional proactive experiences.

PERSONALITY TRAITS OF THE IN-HOME THERAPIST

A review of the literature shows that the in-home practitioner should have certain personality traits. In the field of occupational therapy, Steinhauer (1995) points out that independence, flexibility, adaptability, and ingenuity are required personality traits for those working in-home. He explains that independence is important for the therapist because "there is limited on-site supervision or peer contact in home health relative to institutional settings, so emergencies, conflicts between patients and their families, and tensions with other staff members must be handled independently" (p. 9). Bell (1998) states that "being flexible in an appropriate way to the uniqueness of each home environment, and the lifestyles of those people living together under the same roof, is an essential part of being able to respond therapeutically to the circumstances and needs of patients being cared for at home" (p. 93). The need for adaptability is explained by Bell (1998) in his observation that "to be supportive by demonstrating a willingness to adapt to the pace and routine of the patient and family's domestic life has become a necessary prerequisite to any later discussion about the art therapy" (p. 93).

We often see these personality traits work together under certain demanding circumstances. For example, if the therapist encounters unpleasant home conditions and disrupting distractions such as sudden visitors, calls, and interruptions by other family members during the therapeutic session, the therapist must respond in a positive therapeutic manner. In those situations, the therapist's ingenuity is called upon to continue effective treatment. Lindblad-Goldberg et al. (1998) point out that the in-home therapist must try to find out how to transform those distractions into moments of family competence. A sense of humor and wittiness are useful under these unpredictable circumstances. Lindblad-Goldberg et al. (1998) also argue that the therapist needs to show a willingness to work with the entire family unit. An in-home therapist would be able to:

> . . . first notice and comment positively on any features in the home that demonstrate the family's pride, beliefs, or uniqueness (e.g., family pictures, paintings, decorations, pets, etc.). Thinking about what he or she would want an outsider to notice when first coming into his or her home is a good place for the therapist to start. (Lindblad-Goldber et al., 1998, pp. 92-93)

THE THERAPEUTIC RELATIONSHIP AND THE HOME ENVIRONMENT

In the hospital setting, the patient and his or her family recognize the therapist as an authority figure. In the home environment, a different set of power/controlling relationships (Kunstaetter, 1988) exist. The therapist's position may be less authoritarian and this enables the therapist to create a more intimate and/or social relationship with the family.

The home environment may change the patient-therapist relationship both positively and negatively. Lindblad-Goldberg et al. (1998) discuss proximity and distance in the relationship between the therapist and the client's family. They oppose the assumption that familiarity will decrease the impact of professional interventions. They acknowledge that there is some risk that the therapist may become involved in a family's dysfunctional pattern and absorb the emotions, communicative patterns, and culture of the client's family but they do not see it as largely negative. Since a serious illness or disability affects all family members, it is important for a home-based art therapist to understand and enter family dynamics (Bell, 1998). Family therapy, primarily based on system theory, focuses on altering transactions among family members. The in-home art therapist can incorporate some of these techniques during an art therapy group/family session. Bell (1998) claims that "the skill of the domiciliary art therapist lies in maximizing the opportunities that the home can offer. If this means involving, to a greater or lesser degree, the patient's loved ones, and this may include the family pet, then we must be encouraged to feel confident in widening our approach" (p. 100). A biopsychosocial assessment, which deals with family relationships and social contexts as well as a client's physiology and physical/mental functions (Lindblad-Goldberg et al., 1998) can be administered by an art therapist. They argue that macroassessment (resources of the family and community) and microassessment (symptoms, needs, and strength of the client in addition to his or her historical information) give strength to treatment.

PARADIGM SHIFT IN GERIATRIC CARE AND HOME-BASED ART THERAPY

The biomedical model is explained as the presence of balance or unbalance in a physiological system. Longino and Murphy (1995) explain that the biomedical model separates a human being into mind and body, that it denies an interrelationship between them, and assumes that repairing a body is analogous to fixing a machine. This model has been fundamental in medicine and has a great influence on how doctors comprehend the human body. However, some see it as a limited model. They consider this model very limited since it is adaptable only for a single and clearly identifiable illness, when the elderly usually have multiple and chronic maladies (Longino & Murphy, 1995). Some gerontologists believe that the biomedical model should be replaced with other more holistic models. Williams and Hadler (1983) are two of the most influential figures that promote a paradigm shift in geriatric care. They point out that elderly patients often present with several chronic diseases, many of which are irreversible and incurable, and that treatment should be on modifying the discomfort or disability. Friedan (1993) calls it "a paradigm shift from cure." Another important relevant figure is Robert Butler, who, in an interview with Friedan (1993), emphasized mental health care and psychotherapies for the elderly. He commented, "When you take the functioning of older persons seriously, you can improve their quality of life from even modest changes as opposed to dramatic high-tech 'cures'" (p. 422).

Gibson (1994) appears to be the first art therapist who strongly advocated art therapy for the homebound elderly, supporting the healing quality of art. In art therapy, "their treatments address the problem, develop coping skills, combat depression, enhance quality of life, or prepare the patient for death if that is imminent" (p. 43). With only medical and not psychological support, Gibson explains; "the shortcomings of family members become more evident; complaining and bickering may occur on a daily basis. Even the kind words and acts of loving caregivers add weight to the mounting guilt a patient feels because of his or her dependence and debilitation" (p. 44). In addition, the homebound elderly may feel depressed because of their physical disability and the social stigma attached to the label of "homebound frail elderly." Gibson (1994) presents general treatment goals for this homebound population. Those goals are to:

- Combat depression, report suicide ideology
- Identify unexpressed fear
- Sharpen problem-solving techniques (experimenting with creative solutions to art problems, and transfer of these to other life situations)
- Improve mood
- Assist patient to reconcile living with chronic, physical illness or extreme body losses
- Provide a comfortable level of trust for discussions on sexuality

• Address unresolved family conflicts that impact on patient well-being
• Learn new coping mechanisms (p. 46)

Taking all this background information into consideration, the authors initiated a plan to provide service for the elderly homebound. In the cases that follow, principles of therapies allied with art therapy were considered. In both situations the therapist entered the home with sensitivity in order to determine the needs of the client and support of the family unit. The authoritarian role, often given to therapists in institutions, was abandoned for more proactive, flexible participation centering on the client's strengths. In the first case, various aspects of the client's life were included in her therapy: the home's beautiful surroundings, old photographs, the family pet, the client's caregivers, and the client's innate talent and past successes. In the second situation, self-awareness and self-examination of the art therapist's personality traits in relation to what is desirable for home-care therapy allowed for unique couples' art therapy to unfold. Both cases demonstrate the complexities and possibilities of treatment.

CASE STUDIES

These case studies were conducted under the auspices of a nonprofit, community-based agency that provided various nonmedical services to help disabled residents stay in their home. The agency never had an art therapist until the first author's one-year internship began. The agency's intention is to improve the homebound residents' quality of life.

Case Example: Mrs. J

Mrs. J, a 73-year-old resident suffering from osteoarthritis, scoliosis and osteoporosis, became homebound several years ago. Surgery was not available to her because of her frailty. Other medical problems included high blood pressure, hypothyroid, prolapsed uterus, and gastroenteritis.

Surrounded by beautiful nature, Mrs. J lived in the top floor of a small barn; the ground floor was a garage. Her 50-year-old son, who took her to doctors and shopped for her, lived next door. Her 32-year-old daughter lived locally with her boyfriend. Both of her children were unmarried and did not have children.

Art was especially important for Mrs. J, who had received a one-year scholarship to study fine art when she was younger. After brief employment in the art field, she continued with painting as a hobby; however, that discontinued when she raised her family. Mrs. J's background indicated promise that art activities could refresh her life; she needed encouragement to resume. Mrs. J had sufficient motor skills to paint.

After the first meeting, Mrs. J explained her long-term artistic experiences and showed some of her artwork. The therapist explained the in-home art therapy approach, a client-driven program focused on maintaining a resident's quality of life, in spite of physical decline. Future sessions were scheduled.

Therapy goals for Mrs. J were:

- To express feelings,
- To explore methods of interacting with others,
- To improve/maintain a quality of life through the physical and social changes of her later years,
- To enhance the relationship with her family members including her son, daughter, and ex-husband, and,
- To enjoy the creative process.

Process

During the first sessions, Mrs. J and the therapist painted flowers that were arranged in a vase. The media was watercolor (her favorite), on postcard-sized paper she offered. Mrs. J painted a hydrangea, while the therapist chose a different flower. Mrs. J completed the picture of the hydrangea. Later, she added a bee (see Figure 6-1). More time was allotted in later sessions because Mrs. J wanted time for conversation. She said she could create two or three pictures as homework, which the therapist encouraged her to do. Mrs. J began to paint daily and reported that she even started painting late at night because she could not sleep.

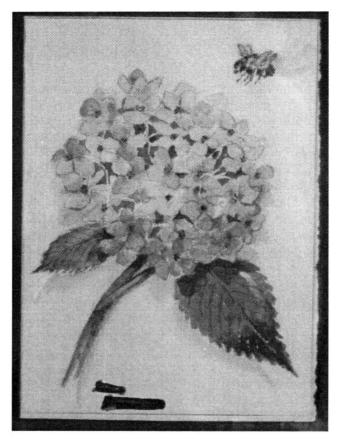

Figure 6-1.

Dialogue during one discussion included the question "Who would you like to send the beautiful postcards you created to?" Mrs. J mentioned one friend, an artist, she no longer saw. This provided an opportunity to talk about friends. Other dialogue invited Mrs. J to discover symbolic meanings in her artwork. For example, when she painted the pictures of her dry flowers and a wooden bird with a metal pot (see Figure 6.2), the therapist asked a question: "If you could be one of the subjects in the picture, which would you like to be?" Mrs. J explained that she would like to be a bee (of which there were two swarming around the flowers) because they can move about freely. She said that she also liked the bird. The therapist asked her to give a title to the picture, and she entitled it a "Metal Pot."

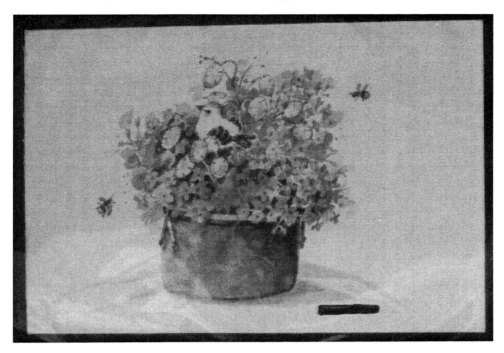

Figure 6-2.

Although focus in discussion was often on the feelings each painting conveyed, Mrs. J asked the therapist to criticize her work and comment on aesthetics, as well. In a picture of a winter landscape, Mrs. J painted an old house from a photograph and added herself and her companion, "Kitty," (a cat) into the picture. Mrs. J and the therapist identified the opened door, the lights inside the house, the particular moment that evening, and the technique used to accomplish her art. A discussion of the warmth of family life followed with descriptions of her early family and their old house. The therapist and Mrs. J discussed writing notes for each piece of art and making a portfolio to contain them. Mrs. J wrote about the subjects in the pictures and how they were related to her. Mrs. J's expanding art activities were facilitated by gifts of art materials from her two children. Mrs. J's daughter gave her watercolor painting paper and a beautiful portfolio; her son bought colored construction paper and picked flowers to use as a model for her pictures.

As therapy progressed, Mrs. J related her encounters with men and her unhappiness. She had two relationships with two men before she married. Painful memories were still revived on St. Patrick's Day, since one old boyfriend had an Irish background. Her marriage, also painful, ended because of her husband's affair with another woman. Mrs. J believed her relationship with her ex-husband influenced her unmarried children and explained that her daughter also had misfortunes in relationships. Mrs. J expressed guilt about her children's education since neither completed college. Some family issues were difficult to deal with since family members never participated in the sessions; however, family was a major issue of discussion, along with her artwork.

With encouragement from her children and the agency, Mrs. J showed dramatic development as an artist. She started spending a great deal of time creating complicated and well-refined pictures.

Discussion

Mrs. J started watercolor painting and produced creative and skillful artworks. She also showed interest in new media and completed a beautiful mosaic. Art became part of her life again; it was recognized by her service agency and family.

The therapist utilized various techniques based on the goals of her therapy. As the regular sessions continued, Mrs. J felt comfortable talking with the therapist about physical pains, negative feelings about her aging, heartbreaking experiences, and family problems. She painted objects that originally belonged to her parents and grandparents. Through painting those objects, Mrs. J reminisced about her family of origin and the beauties in nature that she always loved and admired. Mrs. J showed enthusiasm, motivation, and ambition as she created her portfolio, explored her artistic style, and painted during sleepless nights. Her quality of life changed by retrieving her lost art. Although Mrs. J's children never participated in the sessions, the in-home art therapy provided opportunities to strengthen the relationship between Mrs. J and her children; her artwork became a topic of conversation, and her children supported it by providing art materials and finding models for her pictures.

Professionals who work with the elderly are called upon to examine their perceptions of older clients because a therapist's images about disabilities and aging may directly affect their client's self-esteem.

During art therapy sessions, Mrs. J provided art technique instruction to the therapist who showed his willingness to learn and be taught by someone in a weakened physical condition. This kept a focus on the client's strengths, which embodies a general shift in geriatric care. Older people who are institutionalized generally have few of these opportunities. In the home, Mrs. J read magazines that provided current information, provided gifts independently, and helped others by giving advice. Mrs. J, with assistance from home care services, was able and encouraged to connect to the larger, outside world.

Case Example: Mr. and Mrs. M

Mr. M is a 69-year-old man who is being cared for by his wife in their house because of the debilitating effects of his Alzheimer's disease (AD). He stopped working as a pharmacist five years ago; his wife left her job as an art teacher to look after him. Mr. M. had been taking medication (Aricept®) for six months; the medication, however, did not improve his cognitive impairment. Since then, his regimen has consisted only of vitamins and a baby aspirin daily.

The genetic predisposition of AD was seen in Mr. M's family background, except for his father, who is 94 years old and still physically healthy. The father lives with Mr. and Mrs. M in the same household. Mrs. M is the sole caretaker of both her husband and her father in-law since other family members live far away.

Mr. M does not have any significant physical problems, but AD has affected his cognitive functioning resulting in limited conversation with no deep complexity. Perseveration is a common symptom and a behavioral change that is readily observed. For example, Mr. M repeatedly turned over a hand-held napkin when at the kitchen table.

Weekly, 60-80 minute in-home art therapy sessions were provided for Mr. & Mrs. M. Interventions were aimed at improving the relationship between the couple rather than directly at Mr. M's symptoms. Relationship-focused art therapy for individuals with dementia and their families assumes that the psychological problems of neurocompromised patients, which stem from estrangement, burden, chronic sorrow, result from inappropriate family interactions and dysfunctional coping methods (Johnson & McCown, 1997). Therefore, family therapy art interventions to improve communicative patterns were considered when developing goals. The goals were:

- To enhance the clients' quality of life throughout the process of the disease
- To help the clients understand the reality of the changed family situation and help implement coping skills
- To facilitate communication by providing a nonverbal and visual tool
- To provide the joy of creating artwork and encourage the client and family members to have a meaningful and enriching activity

Process

During the first half of each session over a 10-month period of time, the therapist structured two regularly scheduled activities and one longer art project. The therapist called the two initial activities warm-up exercises, as they were conducted at the beginning of a session. The warm-up helped the clients to feel relaxed. The activities were Visual Conversation (VC) and Squiggle Game (SG); both were used for assessment and treatment as well as relaxation and enjoyment.

In the visual conversation activity (Liebmann, 1986), each participant (two or more) picks up one crayon or marker and starts drawing without talking. The other(s) respond(s) to it in silence. They respond to each other's line/drawing back and forth until the therapist signals to stop. It is not easy for an individual with AD to follow rules (for instance, Mr. M often interrupted the activity by asking, "What's that?" "What is that supposed to be?"); however, the activity is useful to assess the individual's cognitive ability and ways of interacting with others.

The Squiggle Game was designed and studied by D.W. Winnicott (Winnicott, 1971). This therapeutic technique has gained wide attention in art therapy (Zingler, 1976; Simon, 1978). It is usually used with children; however, the technique is adaptable to various populations with some modifications. In the original SG, the therapist imagines a little squiggle (with closed eyes) before drawing it on the paper. Then he asks the client to convert it into a picture. Next the client puts down a squiggle and the therapist changes it in to a picture. During the game, the therapist frequently asks the client about her or his picture.

In the sessions with Mr. and Mrs. M, the therapists adapted these games as drawing for communication. The therapist asked Mr. M to make a picture from a squiggle created by his wife. Mr. M had difficulty working with the shapes drawn by his wife but he could draw lines that related to the shape. When his wife made pictures from his squiggle, he showed obvious enjoyment by his smiles and laughter.

The therapist introduced different media and various activities such as printing, rubbing, magazine photo collage, a town-map making, mandala art, play dough sculpture, etc. Among them, play dough was the most useful media to provide enjoyment to the couple. By using the back and forth modality of the VC project, they passed the dough to reform the shape that was created by other.

After working with the clients for more than three months, therapeutic goals shifted to a strength-based approach aimed at promoting Mr. M's independence and Mrs. M's insight into their changed relationship. The therapist realized that the VC activity had promoted a new, viable relationship as a result of their mutual engagement. Various media and art forms, such as a box, large paper (mural), scroll, and ball were added in the VC activity. Unique and creative adaptations, such as a paper dish mask, a paper tablecloth costume, and foam board printing were also implemented. These product-centered activities were easily completed since they were based on the client's ability and his strength to work within the context of the VC activity.

The plain gift box was the first media introduced for adaptation of the applied VC activity. The box allowed drawing on various sides and on the inside. Following the box project, the therapist implemented a mural project. The large paper size changed not only the clients' visual expressions but also their physical movements. The paper was as large as the dining table forcing the couple to stand up to work; they swung their arms in a large circular motion. They moved together and apart and enjoyed the physical activity. As a follow-up, the therapist utilized the rolled paper (18" x 10') for the scroll project. Their homework, to unroll and work on the scroll, became a challenge that took three sessions to complete. In conjunction with the scroll project, the therapist introduced a paper ball with macaroni inside it. The clients decorated it with the markers and used the VC modality. This project included a variety of stimulating experiences for both participants.

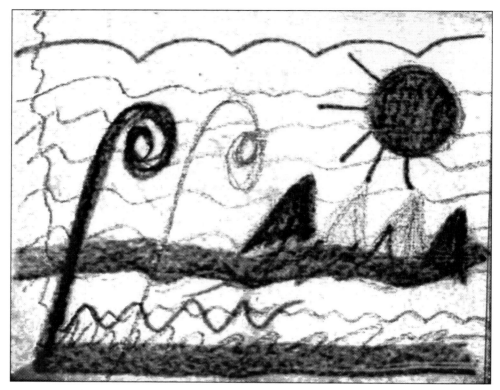

Figure 6-3.

Discussion

In the first Visual Conversation, Mr. and Mrs. M. drew a picture (Figure 6-3). Mr. M started drawing with a purple vertical wave line in the left side. Mrs. M stroked a bold red line on the bottom of the drawing. Mr. M repeatedly drew a horizontal wave line after her drawing. The picture allowed the therapist to understand Mr. M's cognitive impairment and provided a glimpse into the couple's relationship. When Mrs. M drew a spiral line, Mr. M traced it with his purple marker; then he copied it on the right side. In the same way, the sun and small mountain were drawn together. He did not appear confused when following and imitating what his wife did in the drawing.

Another joint drawing was made in the next session. Mr. and Mrs. M had quickly learned how they could communicate with each other by mutual drawings. First, Mr. M. drew a long snake-like black shape; then his wife created a design in the inside of the shape. Again, Mr. M started following his wife's direction by drawing the same kind of stripes. When she put two zigzag lines in the shape, he followed with many wave lines. She gradually understood his ability to follow her direction and together they completed the picture. She did not finish her next strokes in order to let him complete them. She began to test his responses with her art making.

By the sixth session, Mr. and Mrs. M seemed to have developed collaboration through the Visual Conversation. Mr. M always drew first beginning with a large outline; then Mrs. M drew, leading him to follow her direction. Mrs. M told the therapist that continuously making scribbles frustrated her so she began to create figurative pictures. The drawing in Figure 6-4 was created during the sixth session. First, Mr. M drew three circles with a red crayon. This shape was complicated compared to the wavy lines drawn in previous sessions. Mrs. M imagined a snowman giving nonverbal direction to her husband. The picture has a combination of two colors, and all elements became united.

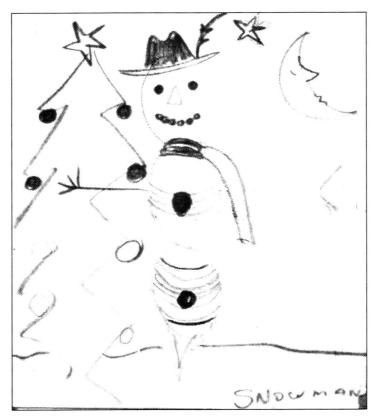

Figure 6-4.

On one occasion, their second son, who visited his parents for Thanksgiving Day, participated in the art therapy session. In this mandala art project, the therapist went first and drew a large circle in the center; he then asked the family to draw lines and shapes in the inside or outside of the circle, all participating simultaneously. Mr. M chose a dark green; Mrs. M chose a light green, and their son chose pink as his color for the drawing. When they finished, the therapist initiated a discussion about the experience and their observations of the artwork. Mrs. M and their son saw that Mrs. M's drawing showed order with rigidity and that Mr. M drew lines only within the circles and did not try to connect. The son found the experience helpful as he had not been able to do anything with his father since the illness prohibited normal interaction. He also felt he communicated with his father in a nonverbal way and was emotionally affected by this session. In addition, he understood what his mother had been trying to tell him about her experiences. They titled their mandala drawing as a "Spinning Wheel."

Eventually, two observations became clear. Mr. M responded to basic geometric lines and shapes quickly, while it took time for him to respond to more complicated shapes. Mr. M showed his frustration by shaking his marker in the air. The shapes and lines he responded to without any sense of frustration were mostly straight lines, circles, rectangles, etc. The second issue was more surprising. In the VC with Mr. M, the therapist copied the way Mr. M drew by tracing his lines or making like ones on the paper. The therapist's imitation sometimes caused Mr. M to give up his imitating and start his own distinct drawing. Later, the therapist encouraged Mrs. M to do the same. Perhaps she could communicate with her husband in this way as well.

During one session the therapist drew a happy face and a sad face in that order. Mr. M immediately responded to the sad face by asking; "Is he sad? It looks like sad to me." He added hair to the face and traced the line of the mouth. At his wife's request, Mr. M wrote her first name on the paper. From this experience, Mrs. M believed that her husband's reactions to those two emotions were still intact. Later, she drew faces during her drawing interaction with him.

Mrs. M reported her observation of the interaction between Mr. M and the therapist. She noticed that prompting Mr. M to respond during the VC was helpful because her husband would lose attention and get confused as to when it was his turn in the conversation. Mrs. M also gained insight into her husband's dependence upon her. She wondered whether her husband could work with others when she was absent. The therapist accepted her suggestion and worked on the next project with Mr. M after she left the room. Mr. M was calm when she was gone and responded positively to the therapist's drawing. This allowed Mrs. M to review and reevaluate Mr. M's need for her constant care.

The media were always important elements of therapeutic art activities because they were related to the client's functional level and therapeutic goals. In the box project, it was noted that in over six visual communication warm-ups, Mr. M never started drawing on different sides of the box by himself. The media was useful to assess the client's flexibility in adjusting to this new medium.

Mr. and Mrs. M successfully completed two large murals. During the discussion, both stated they received satisfaction from this project. The freedom allowed exploration of a new artistic sense and renewed physical energy.

In the scroll project, Mr. M surprised his wife and the therapist by showing his creative drawing and enthusiasm. The scroll included lines he had never created before. It also contained less tracing lines or waves, suggesting that he had some increased independence. The scroll was a document of Mr. and Mrs. M's long journey at working collaboratively; it provided a forum to talk about their previous work. In each session, everyone discussed what had already been drawn before they began new art making. This large artwork and long-term effort enhanced good feelings when it was complete and the entire length of the scroll was seen. Each was surprised by what they had achieved. Mr. M smiled when the therapist applauded his accomplishment. The scroll project had required the clients to walk around the table and stand next to each other, sometimes closely while drawing. During usual art-making sessions they faced each other sitting on opposite sides of the table. The shift of the clients' location during the session allowed physical closeness while developing a new communicative skill.

In the first session of the ball project, Mr. M was overstimulated by this new media and could not decorate it freely (he stuck to drawing the same area and traced it over and over again). The next time, everyone played with the ball before decorating it to become accustomed to handling the media. Playing with the ball gave the couple enjoyment.

Mr. M said "It makes me feel happy." After playing, Mr. M contributed extensively to the decoration. Perceived success in this project led to implementing the mask-making, costume-making, and print-making project.

All art activities sought to enhance the clients' potential for developing communication skills, despite cognitive deterioration. Indeed, the couple did develop communication skills that seemed to please both of them. It was hoped that Mr. M would become more interactive with his environment using acquired communication skills to prevent orderly further deterioration. This approach was also important for Mrs. M because cut-off communication with her ill husband could jeopardize her mental health as well.

These therapeutic art activities displayed the reality of the client's cognitive disease, which had been too painful for his caregiver to recognize. After the initial session, Mrs. M wrote a letter to the service agency and to the therapist. She said she had been depressed after the initial session since she came to recognize Mr. M's severely limited cognitive function and the reality of her living situation as a wife of an Alzheimer's disease victim. The letter validated the therapist's belief that working with the family unit was a helpful service.

The Visual Conversation (VC) activity was appropriate because it encouraged Mr. M's understanding of his wife's visual message. The connections between two different lines indicated that they started communicating with each other again after they had lost the ability for meaningful verbal communication for several years. His wife related that he had asked whether "Chinwa" (his version of the therapist's first name, Shinya) was coming every morning. Their son, who participated in one session, told his mother that he was surprised that he had successful communication with his father through the art activity. These therapeutic gains occurred where the clients felt the most comfortable and secure—at home.

CONCLUSION

Although underdeveloped, art therapy services for the elderly homebound do exist. By using theory from art therapy and allied professions, an art therapist can develop goals and objectives that enhance the quality of life for the homebound person. The domiciliary therapist can provide effective interventions by using his or her own approaches, techniques, creativity, and imagination. The strength of the family unit and home is a resource from which relationships can be understood and utilized as the underpinnings for treatment.

The home setting gives the art therapist a place to be inventive, and in this new era of short-term treatment, it provides the clinician with the opportunity to become involved in long-term care situations. Art therapists, who might enjoy challenges with unwritten rules and mostly uncharted territory, may find home care, with its holistic possibilities, a place to develop new skills and express creativity. They can provide clients with psychological services so vitally needed and often overlooked. Additionally, home-based care offers the art therapist the opportunity for program development. Presently, there is no guide for instituting an effective home-based program, so procedures and the key elements of practice are yet to be developed.

The authors found the experience of home-based care to be satisfying and rewarding and believe in its possibilities. Since funding for research has been a major obstacle, research models for evaluation are limited. Self-report by the families and the agency provided the feedback and encouragement to suggest that more art therapy should be included as a home-based service.

AUTHOR'S NOTE

This article is based on Sezaki's master thesis at Hofsra University, Hempstead, New York. His mentor, Dr. Joan Bloomgarden, was the thesis advisor.

Correspondence concerning this article should be addressed to Shinya Sezaki, 4-21-14, Haijima-cho, Akishima-shi, Tokyo 196-0002, Japan, Email: s_sezaki@hotmail.com and Dr. Joan Bloomgarden, 9 White Deer Court, Huntington, NY 11743, E-mail: cprjsb@hofstra.edu

REFERENCES

Atchley, R. (1987). *Aging: Continuity & change.* Belmont, CA: Wadsworth Publishing Company.

Bell, S. (1998). Will the kitchen table do?: Art therapy in the community. In M. Pratt and M. J. M. Wood (Eds.), *Art therapy in palliative care: The creative response* (pp.88-101). New York: Rutledge.

Friedan, B. (1993). *The Fountain of age.* New York: Simon & Schuster.

Gibson, G. L. (1994). Make art therapy a reality for the homebound. *The Journal of Long-Term Home Health Care: Pride Institute, 13*(3), 43-47.

Johnson, J. and McCown, W. (1997). *Family therapy of neurobehavioral disorders: Integrating neuropsychology and family therapy.* New York: The Haworth Press.

Kerr, C. C. (1999). The psychosocial significance of creativity in the elderly. *Art Therapy: Journal of the American Art Therapy Association, 16*(1), 37-41.

Kunstaetter, D. (1988). Occupational therapy treatment in home health care. *The American Journal of Occupational Therapy, 42*(8), 513-519.

Liebmann, M. (1986). *Art therapy for groups: A handbook of themes, games, and exercises.* Cambridge, MA: Brookline Books.

Lindblad-Goldberg, M., Dore, M. M., & Stern, L. (1998). *Creating competence from chaos: A comprehensive guide to home-based services.* New York: W.W. Norton & Company.

Longino, F. C. & Murphy, J.W. (1995). Paradigm strain: The old age challenge to the biomedical model. In M. M. Seltzer (Ed.), *The impact of increased life expectancy: Beyond the gray horizon* (pp.193-212). New York: Springer Publishing Company, Inc.

Melcher, J. (1988). Keeping our elderly out of institution by putting them back in their home. *American Psychologist, 43*(8), 643-647.

Simon, E. (1978). Drawing games: In art therapy with children. *American Journal of Art Therapy, 17*(3), 75-84.

Steinhauer, M. J. (1995). Home health practice: Consideration for the practitioner. In The American Occupational Therapy Association, Inc., *Guidelines for occupational therapy practice in home health* (pp. 9-14). Bethesda, MD: The American Occupational Therapy Association, Inc.

Williams, M. E. & Hadler, N. M. (1983). Sounding board: The illness as the focus of geriatric medicine. *New England Journal of Medicine, 308*(22), 1357-1360.

Winnicott, D. W. (1971). *Therapeutic consultation in child psychiatry.* New York: Basic Books.

Zingler, R. G. (1976). Winnicott's squiggle game: Its diagnostic and therapeutic usefulness. *Art Psychotherapy, 3*(3-4), 177-185.

Chapter 7

A GRANDMOTHER'S GROUP: ART THERAPY WITH GRANDMOTHERS RAISING ADOLESCENT GRANDCHILDREN

Eileen P. McGann

Current research indicates that the number of grandparents who serve as the primary caregiver for their grandchildren is rising at an unprecedented rate (Bryson & Casper, 1999; Caputo, 1999; Minkler, Roe, & Price, 1992). Many grandmothers have assumed responsibility of caring for their grandchildren as a means of preventing these children from being placed in foster care and away from the family. Often they are living in economic, emotional, and physical hardship. These very special groups of women clearly have a great need for emotional and social support, which most often does not occur in their daily lives (Kennedy & Kennedy 1980; Vardi & Buchholz, 1994). This article looks at the potential of group art therapy as one way to provide therapeutic support and intervention along with encouraging social interaction and emotional support for grandmothers raising adolescent grandchildren.

TREATMENT FACILITY

I work for the Jewish Board of Family and Children's Services in a day treatment program with inner-city adolescent girls and their families. The girls who attend this program have been referred from a variety of sources, including the Board of Education, special education committees, hospitals, residences, and community mental health centers. This voluntary day treatment program, open year-round, provides mental health services and special education classes. Girls and their families make a commitment to wanting treatment in order to be part of this program.

When I began working with adolescent girls and their families in 1986, most of these girls lived with one biological parent. It was an unusual circumstance when a child lived only with a grandparent. This phenomenon has changed considerably over the years. Children living with grandparents as primary caregivers are no longer a rare occurrence. Today, more and more grandparents, particularly grandmothers, are taking responsibility for their children's children. This shift in family dynamics has impacted the nature of clinical work nationwide. Clearly, from personal observation in my work with adolescent girls, the shift in these family relationships impacts all members of the family and brings with it a new set of considerations for the therapist in planning treatment goals and interventions. In addition to the ongoing family meetings, the implementation of a grandmother's art therapy group was proposed as a forum in which to address the growing needs of this special group.

PROFILES OF GRANDMOTHER CARETAKERS

Current research indicates that there is an unprecedented rate at which grandparents have become the primary caregivers for their grandchildren. In 1970, there were 2.2 million children living with their grandparents; in 1993 this number rose to 3.4 million (Caputo, 1999). The United States Bureau of Census revealed that 3.7 million children lived with their grandparents in 1994, and a 1996 report by Kornhabet (as cited in Caputo, 1999) indicated that there were as many as seven million grandparents and grandchildren living together. These numbers clearly point to a rapid shift in the family constellations in our society, of grandparents living with and caring for their children's children. Minkler, Roe, and Price (1992) indicate that the precedence of grandparents raising grandchildren exists across all ethnic groups, yet there is a higher percentage in the Hispanic (5.8%) and African/American (12%) communities (U.S. Bureau of the Census, 1991).

This phenomenon, though a reality in many families, defies the natural order of things. The flow of the life cycle has changed. These women, mostly at or near retirement age have the challenge of raising children again. The circumstances that have led them to being in charge of raising their grandchildren are typically devastating events. Reasons for this dramatic change have been attributed to a number of factors including: parental neglect; abuse; HIV/AIDS; drug involvement; incarceration; death of parent; divorce; and the physical or emotional illness of a parent (Bryson & Casper, 1999). Any one of these factors places the grandparent in a difficult position, and these traumas impact the families greatly. The grandmothers may be in the throes of coping with devastating losses concerning their own children's circumstance. If the death of the parent is the precipitating factor in a grandparent assuming care of his/her grandchild, the loss may be profoundly felt by the surviving family members. In instances where the parent is living, there is often an uncertainty whether or not this parent will return or intermittently appear in the lives of the child and grandparent. This precarious situation, laden with all sorts of potential ramifications, can be devastating to the rest of the family. The anticipation of the parent returning can interfere with any sense of ongoing solidarity or security (Brown-Standridge and Floyd, 2000).

Grandparents can experience guilt and anguish, often along with defensive denial about their own adult children's inability to parent. With increased responsibility and the physical demands of rearing young children, these older women are at risk for greater health complications. Minkler, Roe, and Price (1992) indicate that while physical health and economic situations are affected, the greatest strain on these grandparents is the emotional tension that they endure. The grandchildren they will care for came to them having suffered their own trauma in the loss of a parents, and sometimes additional traumas. Many of these grandchildren are angry and confused by what life has presented them and what they have endured. Clearly the implications of having experienced such personal losses and traumas will impact a persons' ability to cope. Together they are a newly formed family, a team trying to deal with their own feelings as well as each other's.

"The increased psychological distress observed in grandparents raising grandchildren is of major concern for both the grandparents and the children they are raising. Increased psychological distress is associated with poor parenting and family functioning, negative parent-child interaction, and lower child development competence" (Crnic &

Greenber, 1990, as cited in Kelley, Whitley, Sipe, & Yorker, 2000, p. 313). Kelley et al. (2000) cite Milner (1995) in the relationship between psychological stress, impaired ability to effectively manage children's behavior, and the potential for child abuse and neglect.

Therapeutic Goals

The aforementioned statistics serve to demonstrate national trends and occurrences and were not part of the clinical team's discussions. Clearly, no one working with these families needed statistics to demonstrate the stressors of these grandmothers; these women were tired, overburdened, and overwhelmed. They had already faced crises in regard to their adult children and now were faced with raising upset, emotionally-challenged grandchildren, teenagers at that! Who would not need help?

What could we, as clinicians, hope to offer these women? What supports could we provide to assist them, which in turn could benefit the development and life experiences of this next generation of young women they were raising? These adolescent girls have all experienced feelings of resentment, rage, appreciation, relief, and guilt in response to their life circumstances and toward their absent parent and present grandparent. In addition to services for the adolescent girls, which included whatever viable supports from social services that could be elicited, a support group for grandmothers was needed.

Decreasing psychological stress and offering a program that would support these women was a priority in clinical planning. It was anticipated that a group experience could provide a forum for exchange, social support, and mutual learning. The team decided to offer an art therapy group for the grandmothers in the program. It was assessed that in an art therapy group, where emotional issues could be explored and expressed through the art-making, these women could benefit mentally and emotionally. It was hoped that through the art making experience, these women would find a forum for their feelings and be able to reflect upon the processes, thereby fostering an ability to reflect upon their lives. This process of self-reflection, discovery, and increasing personal awareness, along with an attempt to employ new and alternate ways of relating, is an inherent part of the art therapy process. Additionally, social contacts could be increased among peers experiencing common circumstances in the act of creative process. The commonality among group members could also serve to decrease their sense of isolation and increase pleasure in life through the creative act of making art.

The art therapy group was designed to be time-limited, to offer these very busy women the possibility of making a commitment within a set structure. In the past, personal clinical experience has proven that an ongoing expectation is often experienced, at least initially, as another "task" or burden, and not a place of sanctuary or support. For this reason, it was decided to run an initial group for six weeks for an hour and one half a week. All grandmothers were invited to attend. The art therapist sent letters and follow-up calls were made. It was hoped that the girls would also benefit from the involvement of their grandmothers attending the group.

GRANDMOTHERS IN THE GROUP

Of the eight grandmothers who were invited to participate in the art therapy group, six attended the initial session and four members continued to attend regularly. All of the women were of African-American descent, and ranged in age from their early 60s to late 70s. Three of the four consistent members had one granddaughter in their care, while the fourth grandmother was also raising two younger grandchildren in addition to her adolescent granddaughter. All of the participants had been involved with this treatment program, via their granddaughter attending, for at least six months.

Group Structure and Attendance Patterns

The art therapy group was scheduled to meet once weekly for 90 minutes. The first hour was devoted to art making and the last half hour to clean up and refreshments. A full choice of media was available each week including paints, drawing materials, collage materials, and clay works. Each participant was given a professional size portfolio for her work and an art smock. Refreshments consisted of juice, coffee, tea, cookies, and cake. I made it clear that this group was for the grandmothers only—that this was a time just for them. While the granddaughters tested limits around these boundaries during the first two groups, clear parameters were kept and the private workspace of these adult women guarded. While the group had initially been scheduled for six weeks, by the fourth week the women attending requested that the group be extended. It was arranged to have the group meet for an addition three sessions, totaling nine weeks in all.

I ran this group in an open studio approach. The subject matter, themes in the art, and choice of media were left open for participants to decide. This approach was taken because I felt that these were women whose lives were full and had so many tasks and things that were required of them. The burden of often having to meet the expectations and needs of others was a piece of what I hoped they could explore and move away from. Thus, it would have been a contradiction to impose a set of directives or burden these women with any prescribed task. My approach was to encourage them collectively and individually to explore what was most significant. Interventions were geared toward their individual circumstance and need, and not based upon a predetermined set of expectations from this therapist. In taking this approach, it is common for group members to initially struggle with what to do. Often, when a person has been set in a pattern of doing for others, or living in a reactive manner, there is uncertainty in initially identifying and then asserting one's own needs and preferences. This was the initial response of most group members.

Group Process and Dominant Issues That Emerged

Phase 1: Initial Anxiety and Uncertainty, or "Where do I begin?"
During the first few weeks of the group, members exhibited uncertainty about the art-making process and anxiety in this new situation. Initial indecision and anxiety seemed in part to be related to uncertainty about what direction to take. I purposely did not assign a task for these women to complete or attempt to execute. Again, my feeling was that they have so many things they *must do*, that this would be an opportunity for them to explore and develop what they might *want to do*.

My experience has been that while this initial period of uncertainty and anxiety may be uncomfortable for the participants, ultimately the work and therapeutic process have much more meaning if the messages and images are of the individuals design. I have found that the potential for greater trust and fuller engagement occurs when a set course of treatment, specifically art directives, is *not employed*. Obviously, this is my personal and professional bias, and in such, I feel that the treatment is more genuine.

Group members initially relied upon the art therapist for technical advice, support, and demonstration in their art making, relating to the art therapist as the provider of instruction. As their individual and collective needs and requests were attended to, group member's nurturance needs were attended to. The unspoken dependency desires and support these women experienced were beginning to be addressed in this forum. It was a significant transformation for some of these women to go from the role of sole provider of other's needs, to the one who was on the receiving end of nurturance and support. Only one expectation was set, implied, and at times spoken: that this art therapy group was a forum just for them. The therapeutic goal was that they would be able to use the time and materials for themselves, and that the companionship of other women with similar circumstances would provide a forum for mutual support and exchange.

Phase 2: Issues of Abandonment, or "They left me." Group members explored and expressed issues of abandonment in several ways. When two members did not return after the first group, the four remaining group members projected their anger onto me and held me responsible for their peers not continuing. One group member informed me that it was my "poor planning" and "no understanding of the needs of black women" that caused the decline in group membership. This member also stated, "Black women don't like to paint." She and another member concurred that a knitting group would have been more productive in terms of membership.

These accusations appeared to reflect a sense of hopelessness in my ability to truly understand, support, or be of any help to them. The angry focus on our obvious differences in terms of ethnicity (I am Caucasian) left me wondering if age also would become an issue as I was 25 to 30 years younger than the group members. It has been my experience that when there is such anger and focus on external differences, this rage is based in fear and past experiences of pain. My response to the anger of the remaining group members was to acknowledge their frustration. I concurred that I did not know the first thing about knitting but that I felt art making had little to do with age or race, and that their achievements in the art thus far were a testament to that fact. Furthermore, I agreed that it was disappointing when people left, particularly when you looked forward to their company. I questioned them as to whether the absence of a few might have to do with their life circumstances and not so much about the group or remaining members. I articulated what value the group had to me, and the positive impact they had upon each other thus far. I suggested that they continue to attend and evaluate at the end of the group duration whether or not they would like to continue this or another type of group in the future.

Another woman reacted to the loss of peers feeling personally rejected and abandoned, "I thought we were having fun and they left me." These comments were followed by discussion of her adult children no longer keeping in touch with her, and the impact this significant loss has upon her life. The understanding of this loss was observed in other members nodding their heads in agreement.

While the anger and resentment of a few group members was vented directly toward me, it was hard not to personally feel sad for them in response. The sting of rejection, and the angry pride to not articulate their needs and desires in the moment was clearly painful for them to endure. My therapeutic goal here was to try and help these women identify and articulate the value and investment they were making in this group, and in themselves. Furthermore, I believed that the art-making experience and therapeutic forum would transcend barriers on many levels.

Phase 3: The Arts as a Soothing Experience, or "This is very calming." From the start, despite some initial anxiety from several group members, the soothing quality of the sessions and the art making was observable. Group members expressed appreciation for the quiet, calm atmosphere of the art therapy room. They were surprised and accepting of the space being solely for them and not for the children. The women commented on the plants, sculptures, and paintings that filled the room. The atmosphere was one of genuine work and artistic pursuit, without interruption. Group members demonstrated a desire to participate and connect with other members around the art making. It appeared that in doing so, they were able to move from the place of identified "caregiver/grandparent" to that of "artist." At the beginning, conversations about home dominated, but subsided after the first two weeks; then the women focused more on exploring individual interests, which was reflected in the art-making processes. As silence began to dominate the sessions, members became increasingly absorbed and conversations focused on the practical and aesthetic qualities of their work. One woman began coming to session wearing "an artist's beret." Her observable change in dress was paralleled by her articulated position as "an artist." Value of the art and the experience as soothing was articulated by several participants, with comments such as, "This is very calming, very relaxing," and "I want more art therapy." "I wish I could come here every week, all through the summer. This is a place just for me to be." This last comment was made by the grandmother who initially sat silent and did not participate.

Phase 4: The Value of Companionship and the Mutual Support of Group Members. Initially, there was little overt acknowledgment by these women of the art therapy arena being a "therapy" group. Discussions about weekly life events, the demands on their time, and the toll this took on their energy were the verbal focus during the first two meetings. Group members were eager to share common experiences of family life, the difficulties of commuting to the program, and the challenge of raising teenage girls. Through these shared experiences of common family issues and a need for time for themselves, group members began to form a bond with each other. Additional comments concerned their self-consciousness about participating in an art group. When one member joked about her grandchild being able to draw better than she could, I intervened by observing that it had probably been years since many had been involved in an art program, and that while their grandchildren were still being given this opportunity in school, this now was an opportunity for them as well. I informed the group that one of the 'rules' I impose in the art therapy is to not allow for insults to artwork, including their own. Group members met this with some surprise, yet it was simultaneously accepted and respected. Specific struggles in art and specific comments about developing one's own work would be encouraged, but general insults or teasing about their own or other's efforts would not be allowed. I explained that it was my feeling that if people felt unsafe to make art, this group experience would not have a chance to succeed. The women clearly understood this, and what emerged was 'permission' to participate with a greater sense of safety. This verbal exchange led to a focused involvement in the art making, and group members demonstrated acceptance of their own struggles with genuine support of each other's artistic processes. This was demonstrated in shared materials, common themes in the art, constructive criticism, and recognition of each other's artwork.

Ultimately the group came together around materials and themes in the art. This group cohesion was evidenced in the shared focus of media (all working in clay, and later on, all creating flower drawings in pastel; see photos). Notable was the genuine appreciation for each other's art and encouragement between members to complete their work and display it. The one member who initially did not attempt to create any work and had assumed the role of critical director was challenged by the other women in the group to "stop just sitting there telling everyone what to do and do some yourself!" In letting go of this position, what I perceived as a fear-based stance, afraid to risk exposure or the negative criticism she was projecting onto others, the group met her with acceptance and inclusion. This transformation was remarkable to observe. At no time did other group members directly or indirectly retaliate; rather they embraced her efforts to join with them.

Outside of the group, connections that began in this art therapy group were continued between several members. These women openly discussed their telephone contacts, plans to socialize outside of the group and encouraged other members to join them. Two members in particular maintained close contact and attempted to attend social activities, specifically church-related events that included their granddaughters.

Phase 5: Requests for Continued Art Therapy. The four group members who attended the sessions on a regular basis all requested that the art therapy group be continued for additional meetings. All members were able to bring their artwork to completion and articulate the value of the time and companionship in their lives that the group had provided. These women were able to specifically praise the accomplishments of other members, and talk about the art being a time they looked forward to. One member stated, "I wait all week for this group. I think about what I am going to do on my painting long before I get here." Another woman expressed total surprise when the last session occurred, "I can't believe this is it! I really am going to miss this. Can we paint again next year?" Additionally, it was observed that all members gained a sense of mastery and accomplishment in their individual artwork. I provided all group members with the option to matt and frame their drawings and paintings, as well as to mount the one sculpture that was completed. It was important to me that each member understand the value of her work. I am quite particular with the care and display of artwork, as this message of value and acceptance is a vital part of the art therapy process. In the final group session, each member appeared to embrace the mounting and display of their artwork without reservation.

Individual Notes and Artwork of the Group

In addition to the issues that emerged for the group, I would like to describe and discuss some of the individual issues and artwork of the four women who participated on a regular basis: Mrs. C; Mrs. J; Mrs. K and Mrs. T.

Mrs. C

Mrs. C traveled for two hours on public transportation in her wheelchair in order to attend this weekly art therapy group. This factor in itself speaks of the interest and investment she had in being a member of this group. The struggle of her travel was a major factor in how she initially presented herself to other members of the group. She would arrive late, breathless, and with long detailed account of how trying the journey had been. During the first two sessions, other group members were extremely empathic and sympathetic to her struggle, frequently offering to help her physically and retrieve materials for her to use. With the group's attention focused on her physical struggles, Mrs. C appeared to escalate in her long sighs, moans, and complaints. Additional complaints were typically framed around her individual suffering for the good of her granddaughter or adult children, casting her into the role of a martyr. By the third session however, other group members, all with various challenges of their own, stopped responding to Mrs. C's remarks and sounds.

When group members stopped affirming her verbalizations, and I focused on Mrs. C being in the group for herself, relating to her genuine achievements in art, Mrs. C abandoned the role of a chronic complainer. Mrs. C consistently had difficulty leaving at the end of the group, delaying her completion of work, and prolonging the packing up of supplies. This had both a desperate quality of neediness and of passive aggression, suggesting the extent and depth of her own emotional deprivation.

Strengths in her demeanor and art-making process were also present and observed. Mrs. C was able to abandon a helpless, angry stance in favor of a more productive and ultimately fulfilling position in relation to the art-making process. She was quite self-directed in her choice of media and subject matter, and repeatedly made reference to the planning and thinking about her work between sessions. Careful attention to detail noted in the tempera painting, as well as in the clay work, demonstrated care and value of her self that was explored through the art-making (see Figure 7-1).

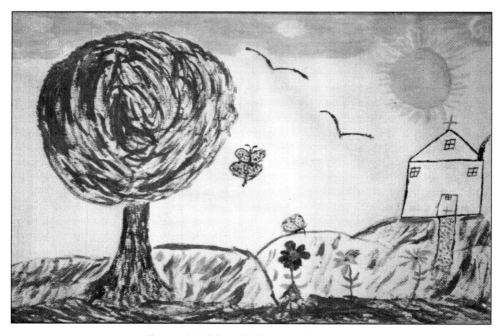

Figure 7-1. Mrs. C's Tempera Painting.

The dominant theme in her artwork related to the role of religion in her life. A clay cross was created to hang at home, and a tempera painting depicts a church she attended as a child. The care that she took in selecting colors, and detailing this piece over several weeks, was reflective of the depth of investment she had in this process. During the painting, Mrs. C openly discussed feeling alone, without the support of extended family, and how she sought consolation and support from her church. Group members responded in kind, noting the importance of religion in their lives as well. Additionally, Mrs. C was invited to participate in a church social activity, along with two other members. The consistent provision of a forum in which she could safely explore and express feelings of anger, isolation, and helplessness and create in the art metaphors for these issues seemed to significantly contribute to her sense of well-being.

Mrs. J

In the initial group, Mrs. J sat and observed the others, but did not engage in any art making herself. She directed others as to what they should do with their artwork, though obviously wanting to be more involved. Her negative stance was confronted by the other group members, who were not willing to tolerate her dictating without risking her own expression. "You just sit there and tell everyone what to do with their work, what about you? Why don't you do something?" This initial negative stance seemed to be a defense against feelings of insecurity and vulnerability. Tentatively, she began to work. Self-conscious about working, she compared her art to that of "my 3-year-old grand," saying he could do better. Her effort to create art and be a part of the group was met with genuine support by other group members. The encouragement she received enabled her to continue.

Following a three-week absence, her return was met with an enthusiastic welcome by the other women. Following the lead of other group members who were working on pastel drawings of flowers, Mrs. J carefully traced, transferred, and completed a bunch of tulips (see Figure 7-2). Pride in this work was noted in her careful approach, the absence of any self-degrading remarks, and the increased focus in her own work. Mrs. J had abandoned the role of dictating to others what they should be doing and had assumed a place as an active participant of the art therapy group.

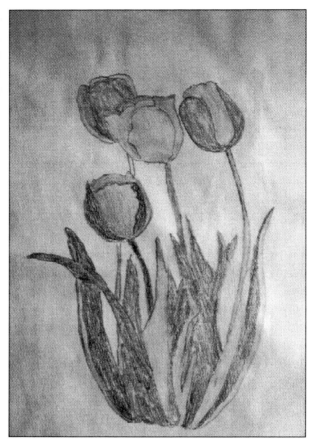

Figure 7-2. Mrs. J's Tulips.

Mrs. J was able to accept affirmation from other group members about her work, and offered in response genuine praise of peer's accomplishment. Surprising to me, in the last group that she attended, Mrs. J asked if the art therapy group could meet all summer. She said that this was the only time she had to herself and that she really wanted a place and time set aside to do something just for herself. Initially, she had rejected the art and asked for knitting, saying that she was going to teach everyone. In the end, she was accepting of and embraced the art. So in this process Mrs. J shifted from feeling that she had to teach and provide for others, to allowing herself to be cared for and provided for in the art therapy group.

Mrs. K

Mrs. K began one tempera painting and completed one flower drawing. In the initial session, Mrs. K looked though books and magazines, uncertain of what to do. Focused on her own review of materials, she interacted minimally with other group members. In the second session, she worked on copying a seascape of an empty boat on a shore. This image seemed to parallel her place in the group. She was significantly confused about details of the structure of the group. She repeatedly asked questions about the meeting times, day of the week, and other basic life knowledge that indicated she was experiencing some confusion.

Mrs. K's artwork demonstrated a capacity for organization, greater than her verbalizations would indicate. She keenly focused on the details of the painting and demonstrated a sensitivity to color. Mrs. K worked in a focused manner to copy the seascape in a realistic way. She easily accepted technical instruction from me, and welcomed the comments from other women in the group.

After an absence from the group, she returned to abandon this painting in favor of working on a pastel flower drawing (see Figure 7-4a), similar to what other women were working on. While it was distressing to have her abandon her own idea, the desire to be more connected with other group members was expressed in her assuming a similar image as the other group members. During work on this final piece, Mrs. K related more to the others, engaged in conversation, and praised the artwork of others. It seemed that the social connection and organizing influence of the art making was the most significant factor for Mrs. K.

Mrs. T

Mrs. T completed two tempera paintings and one pastel drawing during the course of art therapy sessions (see Figures 7-3a and 7-3b). Mrs. T initially appeared oblivious to peers' processes or needs, often interrupting their work or conversations with issues of her own. Seemingly, she had little interest or awareness of the needs of others. This seemed to speak of her own emotional neediness, and desire for my undivided attention; however, as the group progressed, this subsided. As her own needs were being met, through my support, the art-

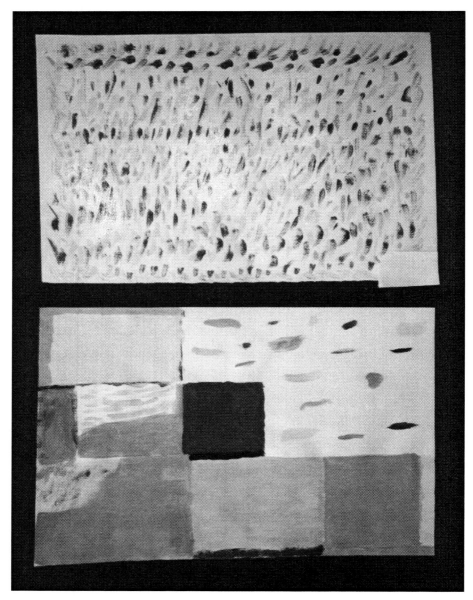

Figure 7-3a/7-3b. Two tempera paintings by Mrs. T.

making processes, and the positive verbal affirmations of her artwork from peers, she was able to extend herself to other women in the group and related in a more socially reciprocal manner. The connections she made in the group extended to her calling others outside of the group for activities at her church and other gathering places.

In terms of her artwork, Mrs. T was self-directed and extremely focused. Her ability to analyze her work was noteworthy; she was able to assess what she liked, what she was not satisfied with, and take the necessary steps to correct it. This planned and methodical approach to her work at times seemed quite contradictory to her impulsive verbal intrusions and occasional physical intrusions, i.e., grabbing materials without looking at others using them. The first piece, a multicolored painting of brush strokes, was executed in a slow and methodical manner. Mrs. T described this work saying, "I just let it flow. I just let it happen." Her second painting, a more structured, though abstract piece, required more planning and mixing of colors. During her work on this, Mrs. T referred to several contemporary art books for reference. She began to come to session wearing "an artist's beret" and her demeanor in the group shifted. The organizing principles employed in this painting carried over into her relationship with others; Mrs. T was less intrusive of others' space, and more tolerant of my attention to other group members.

Her final piece, a pastel drawing of flowers, was the most structured (Figure 7-4b). She worked carefully to create and color these tulips. The result is a realistic image of colorful flowers. This work, in image and in process, connected her with other group members who were also working on pastel flower drawings. In looking at the progression of Mrs. T's artwork, one can see an increased cohesiveness through the art. This paralleled her relationship with others in the group, suggesting increased ego strengthening brought on by the support of the group. Similar to Mrs. K, the art appeared to have a strong organizing effect for Mrs. T.

Mrs. T's connection to the group and investment were evidenced not only in her consistent attendance, but also in her request for a continuation of the group into the next year. When other group members did not return or were absent, Mrs. T responded with anger directed toward me. She projected these feelings of abandonment and rage onto the leader, holding me responsible for a fracture in what I perceived as a special experience for her. Given the space to vent this anger, and with my acknowledgement that it is upsetting when people don't return or value what you do, she continued to attend and ultimately praised the group art therapy experience. First, her anger, and later, her attendance and active participation, was deemed to be a reflection of her desire for increased social support and nurturance. She received this support and affirmation from myself and other group members through validation of her artwork, technical support of supplies, and the art therapy forum itself.

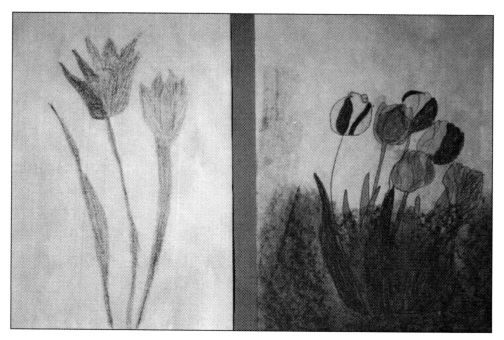

Figure 7-4a. Artwork of Mrs. K.   Figure 7-4b. Artwork of Mrs. T.

In the last group, Mrs. T offered high praise of the group experience, and trust in the art therapist. She told another group member who was debating what to do with a section of her drawing, "Just ask Eileen. She'll tell you—Why she can help you bring a little nothing into something. She'll help you with just the right amount of direction to keep you going on your own and make it work."

SUMMARY

This nine-week grandmother's art therapy group was an enlightening experience for me as an art therapist. In retrospect, while I did not consciously begin the group with set expectations about subject matter and themes, I do realize that I was anticipating that these women would focus on the common experience of rearing grandchildren. While discussion about this did occur in the initial session, and subsequent discussion related to feelings of loss and abandonment by family members, on the whole, the group members moved in another direction. The predominant issues that emerged appeared to be related to the soothing effect the art-making experience provided them as well as the comfort of the support gained through the peer companionship that developed.

These women clearly embraced the calming atmosphere of the art therapy arena and were connected to the art-making experience. Each member of the group contributed to this ambiance developing and existing. Another seemingly significant contributing factor was providing them with a space that was just for them. In guarding their privacy from the interruptions of their grandchildren, who attempted and requested to be part of this group, these women were given an opportunity to begin to identify and pursue individual interests. I do not mean to imply here that more inclusive family work is not warranted— it is. There is, however, tremendous value in allowing these women to care for themselves and be supported in a role other than the family caregiver.

As stated in the group and individual notes, there was a period of time when all four women were working on similar images of flowers. Clearly they were relating and connecting with each other through shared images and materials. The careful drawing and gentle approach in the coloring seemed to reflect a growing care that they were taking in regard to themselves. Most evident to me was the self-soothing quality the art making was providing them in this forum. The vibrant colors seem to speak of the life and growth potential within them.

Through the art making and group experience, these women were able to assess their own desires and means of relating, as seen in the artwork and group discussions. The shift in functioning seems to be reflective of an internal shift in which there was an increased sense of genuine acceptance and pleasure, accompanied by a decrease in stress during this group experience. As these women found a place together, their work collectively and individually became more organized and structured, suggesting that there was also an experience of integration from this group.

The positive effects of this grandmother's art therapy group are evident. While this forum may thus far have been underutilized, the potential for further work exists. As in all family work, when one member is affected, the entire family will often experience ripple effects of the changes. In addition to the benefits noted for these grandmothers, their granddaughters' school performance shifted during this time period. Improved on-time attendance, classroom behavior, and therapeutic milieu encounters were notable. As art therapists, we have a unique opportunity to impact upon the lives of these grandparents and their grandchildren through the therapeutic use of art and group practice. Once again, I am amazed with the healing power of art. I feel fortunate to have been a witness to and part of this experience, and look forward to further groups of this nature.

REFERENCES

Brown-Standridge, M. D., & Floyd, C. W. (2000). Healing bittersweet legacies: Revisiting contextual family therapy for grandparents raising grandchildren in crisis. *Journal of Marital and Family Therapy, 26* (2), 185-197.

Bryson, K., & Casper, L. M. (1999). Co-resident grandparents and grandchildren. In U.S. Department of Commerce, Economics and Statistics Administration, *Current population reports, special studies*, (p. 23-198). Washington, DC: U.S. Government Printing Office.

Caputo, R. (1999). Grandmothers and co-resident grandchildren. *Families in Society: The Journal of Contemporary Human Services,* March- April, 120-126.

Kelley, S. J., Whitley, D., Sipe, T. A., & Yorker, B. C. (2000). Psychological distress in grandmother kinship care providers: The role of resources, social support, and physical health. *Child Abuse and Neglect, 24*(3), 311-321.

Kennedy, J. F., & Kennedy, V. T. (1987). Group psychotherapy with grandparents rearing their emotionally disturbed grandchildren. *Group, 11*(1), 15-25.

Minkler, M., Roe, R. M., & Price, M. (1992). The physical and emotional health of grandmothers raising grandchildren in the crack cocaine epidemic. *The Gerontologist, 32*(6), 752-761.

Vardi, D. J., & Buchholz, E. S. (1994). Group psychotherapy with inner-city grandmothers raising their grandchildren. *International Journal of Group Psychotherapy, 44*(1), 101-121.

Chapter 8

LESSONS FROM ELDERS: ART THERAPY IN A SENIOR APARTMENT COMPLEX

JAN FENTON

Τhis chapter will examine the need and importance of short-term and/or continuing art therapy sessions for a group of female older adults. The group discussed came from various ethnic and cultural backgrounds, most of whom were widowed and living along for the first time in years.

Many urban and suburban cities and towns now provide housing for the population described above, and occasionally offer minimal recreational/social pursuits for interested residents. Socialization is important, especially as one faces a recent loss and a new, more independent lifestyle. Bonding with others, in new circumstances, is vital for lessening of depression in the elderly. It is a time of great loss (health, loved ones, finances); support, or some type of therapy, could truly help. In working with older adults, sensitivity must be used in naming/defining the purpose of such sessions, since there can be a negative reaction to anything that bears the name "therapy." This generation is not used to having others help them solve their problems, but the plain fact is that it *is* therapy, and art therapy works! It works at a deep, meaningful level and can effect change and transition on several levels: enhancing self-esteem, encouraging communication, facilitating expression, respect and bonding with peers, and diminishment of loneliness/isolation.

THE FACILITY

The apartments where this work took place was a newly opened facility for older adults who have the ability to care for themselves

163

without daily assistance. They live independently in their own apartments in approximately 40 units. There were widows, widowers, singles, and a few couples in the residence.

The recreation department in the town offered two days a week of activities for older adults. These were conducted in another part of town, a short drive from the residence. Only a small percentage of residents attended these town-sponsored events. Realizing the need for more services, I offered to do an on-site art therapy group. The director of the apartments was delighted to be offered volunteer help. It was badly needed since all the residents had just moved into the apartments, and were going through a lot of transitions. Though surface pleasantries were exchanged in the hallways and on the elevator, these people really did not know each other.

THE GROUP

Art therapy can be very beneficial to all populations, but it is especially useful for this population as they are in the midst of yet another life change. This transition to senior apartments is much more than just a move from a house to an apartment. Most of the people have some health problems, although they are functioning well on a daily basis. Many of them have experienced wrenching losses of their mates and even children. Some had never lived alone before, going from their parents' homes into marriages. The women attendees were a multicultural and multiracial group. The one thing they all had in common was their advanced age and the move to such a residence. However, each person was a stranger to the other. Attending the group were women from the Bronx, South Carolina, Northern and Southern Ireland, Poland, and a Middle Eastern country. All of the women were widows, except for two. No men attended.

Resistant as this group was to both the thought and the word "therapy," care was taken to introduce these sessions as "art therapy." These simple workshops led to socialization and friendship where none existed, and began to help this group of women to establish a new sense of place. During a series of art therapy sessions, some important breakthroughs in intercommunication took place. Relationships to their new surroundings were also greatly enhanced.

This chapter will encourage and provide suggestions for 12 work-shops. You will note that the beginning sessions seem to have more activities. As a deepening trust developed and along with some confidence in use of materials, the participants were more able to a focus and there was less need to "switch gear." The group sessions took place in a community room within the building. Each session ran for one and a half hours. A flyer advertising the new group was posted in the building lobby and also put in each resident's mailbox.

Session I

At the first session, I introduced myself and then asked each person to reveal a bit about herself using simple facts, like where they were born, grew up, etc. They seemed genuinely delighted to speak and share with each other and interacted well in the group milieu.

For the first activity, they were asked to put their apartment keys on the table. They could either trace the keys or draw them free hand. This activity was very nonthreatening and required little to no artistic ability. Some were daring enough to simply draw a key, others felt safer tracing them, and one woman covered the page with tracings of various keys to make an overall design. Almost everyone chose to color their pictures. Some of the women seemed very timid in the approach to the assignment, while those with some art experience proceeded confidently; no one refused to participate.

Next, we did a puzzle game. On a specially marked piece of puzzle paper (precut and secretly numbered), each person could draw anything she wanted. They could fill it in anyway they wanted–realistic or abstract, or with stripes and polka dots . . . whatever. They had no idea what their odd-shaped piece of paper was to become. It was going to fit together to form a puzzle picture. Everyone chatted and got into the project.

When I asked them to bring their finished piece together, they were surprised to see it all fit together. This was then used as a metaphor to say, "You are all part of this picture of this new life at the apartments." They were very pleased.

The last thing I had them do was to draw a tree–any tree, a tree they especially liked. Unbelievably, or as most art therapists might guess, none of the trees had roots. Their roots had been pulled up for this

probable last move of their lives. One of the women drew a very frag-
ile and disconnected tree, and she did not return to our group. Later I
learned she was struggling with cancer and she died not long after.

Session II

During the second session, I presented them with their finished
work: the puzzle picture was finished and framed to be hung in their
hallway that was noticeably bare of any artwork. We then started with
the day's session. They had been asked to bring a photo, which I
would copy for them on the copying machine. They were not familiar
with the word or concept of collage. Many brought photos of their
deceased husband. One woman had a copy of her deceased husband's
photo, which I then copied. Then she was instructed to look through
magazines and cut out images that represented his life and interests.
"Oh yes, what an outdoor and Mr. Fix-it man he was. He loved the sea
and I must find a picture of a hammer. He was always hammering
away at something." You could see a liveliness about her as she lov-
ingly recalled memories of her husband. Another had a photo of her
living husband. "That's him standing next to some large green garden
plant." She was then asked to see if there were any gardening cata-
logues in which she could find further images of the interests her husband had before he became ill.

One of the ladies had a bunch of photos in her purse that she carried about with her. There was a picture of a baby, perhaps a friend's.
I asked if she would like to do a collage of someone closer to her. (I
had hopes that she might process her husband's death/life in this way,
but she resisted.) "No, I love this baby, I'll do this." She pasted the
copy of the child's photo to the page and she used heart-shaped cookie cutters to outline designs around the page. Another group member
wanted to focus on her grandchildren; she listened and watched the
others but did not go any further. She said she would do hers later in
her apartment. Another had forgotten a photo but she, too, began to
gather ideas for her collage and she talked freely about her husband.
This exercise seemed to be a gentle way of getting into some of the loss
and grief they had experienced. "He was all business. Always thinking
of work. He dressed very nice. I could find some picture of offices or
something like that, couldn't I?" she asked.

As things began to lag in the session, I changed the focus to a neutral one in order to end on a positive note. This time, I introduced the basic shapes exercise of circle, triangle, and squares. I had a batch of assorted shapes cut from cardboard so they could trace or create their own design. They could use just one kind of shape to make a design, or use assorted shapes, or make something realistic or recognizable from the shape. Everyone did the random shapes. One woman made a country cottage, another did a bunch of balloons, and some just layered the shapes in a variety of ways, including overlapping. Then they got interested in using color. I worked alongside the women and did concentric lines inside some of the shapes I had chosen. The woman next to me integrated this idea into her picture with no overt teaching going on, just through her observation. They were remarkable pieces and they all began to notice how each person had the style and color choice of their own.

Near the end of the session, a resident in the house dropped by. After observing for a while she said, "Well you may get angry, but this drawing stuff is not for me." I told her that that was okay and she could visit and go as she pleased and that if she ever wanted to join the group, she would always be welcome. One of the women remarked to her "it is not the work, but being together that is so nice." Another agreed and said, "Even if it is foolish, I like trying new things." Other comments from the group included, "I like to do this–besides, it's relaxing." "Even though I'm not good at this, I like to come to be with everyone." "I like to play with the colors." "Yes, Yes, this is so good, it makes me feel good to come here, to talk together and to color." "It makes my heart happy to be here." (And, of course, as a therapist, it made my heart happy to hear this response.)

Session III

During the next session, not everyone had collage material, so we moved to another focus and did a loosening up exercise–the scribble. They were slightly aghast at the idea of just letting their arm move freely. First, I did a demonstration of the "follow me" scribble. A resident and I both picked out different colors and play a kind of follow-the-leader routine to make our picture on the same paper. Then another resident did the next one with me, and she was the leader that I followed. We then tried to see if we could make any sense out of the image. They were ready to start their own scribble drawing, and glad when I suggested they could add more color, maybe sectioning and delineating things in various ways, using colors. During this exercise they laughed a lot at the beginning. One member said that hers looked like a storm, a hurricane, all busy and swirling. Some were very engrossed in their own work, saying little. Then things became quite relaxed and side conversations were also pursued while working. "Do you think Clinton is handsome?," one said. I was asked if I thought the man on a certain TV show was handsome.

One woman commented with a smile, "I feel like a kindergartner." Another said, "Oh, we never got to do things like this in school. We only learned needle work." Others started to discuss the strictness of their school years.

One woman recalled, "They used a switch on me in school, in Ireland," and she still had the mark on her wrist to prove it. Another commented that her nuns never hit her. Then one of the women mentioned her grandfather who owned a farm. "He would go out on horseback to check up on any lazy workers, and he would carry his whip." One group member worked painstakingly, and with great skill, and filled in her scribble, which became an ordered expanse across the page. She was one who frequently asked to complete her work at home, which meant, to me, that the art therapy was having an impact beyond the sessions.

This scribble warm-up gave them renewed interest in completing the collages that they had started. The gardener's wife had brought in squares neatly cut out from vegetable seed catalogs. Others were finding images from magazines during the session that might be useful. In the meantime, the lady who had remembered her grandfather's strictness was busy drawing Mt. Etna smoking with red lava pouring out. She said, "They were punished for their evil ways." She insisted, "People are evil and have these things happen to them. Whenever these things happen, like disasters, just dig and you'll find they were bad," she said. Some of the women were appalled but it led to a rich discussion. She was asked about good, innocent people who have had bad things happen to them. And the fact that many bad people do not necessarily suffer. It was a fair discussion and everyone seemed to have their say. Perfectly timed, snow started falling quietly, peacefully, shifting our attention to the time. We decided that it was time to stop and have a cup of tea. The director of the facility suggested that we could use the room for a longer period if people wanted to eat their lunches together. The group lingered for 20 minutes after the tea, for conversation.

Session IV

I was beginning to learn that due to memory problems or scheduled doctor appointments, it was not always possible to have a full class.

For this session, one woman arrived late, but proudly brought in a paper with some palm trees sketched on it. She explained that she had done this while watching a show about trees on TV. Another woman brought in her completely reworked scribble drawing that was masterful. I felt some of this work should be displayed, as the group members were very proud of their accomplishments.

Since this was the fourth meeting, I had the attendees review the work they had done. Usually within a group, there is a bit of comparison if one or more of the members are gifted in art. It can also make people somewhat embarrassed about their own work. Care must be taken to point out each person's work with regards to the others feelings. The women seemed pleasantly surprised at the amount and the level of the work they had accomplished.

It was now March, and we went with a calendar theme for that day's session—St. Patrick's Day. The shamrock is an easy and attractive symbol to play with. And as there was to be a St. Patrick's Day party, their work could be part of the décor. Some did shamrocks and some four-leaf clovers. They talked about "luck." One woman even had such a charm on her bracelet. One spoke of converting the pagans, Druids. One of the Irish ladies recalled a story told her as a child about the shamrock and the Trinity. Whatever the religious background, the topic seemed to interest them all.

Shifting gears again, I introduced the idea of wax resist. I did this by demonstrating a crayon drawing that could be watercolored over. Using only the simplest materials, and ones that they were now familiar with, they timidly tried out the technique. Emboldened with gaining some control over the materials, they grew more free and did not feel compelled to work realistically. Their work flowed like the watercolor and became more abstract.

Towards the end of the group, we began talking about having lunch together. One woman offered to make potato pancakes, her specialty. Not one person left; all stayed to have lunch together. Instead of eating up in their apartments alone, they now were indeed socializing. I had hoped this would be ongoing; however, it did not occur again. People were willing to stay for tea, but it seemed that after the art group, they had had enough activity and preferred to return to their apartments.

Session V

Today, I set out to have the group be more spontaneous. Using only crayons or pastels and larger paper, they were first to pick a color. Using their entire arm from the shoulder, they were to draw vertical, horizontal, or circular motions. Then they switched hands, to use their nondominant hand. After that loosening-up exercise, they were to scribble on a new piece of paper and see what emerged.

They were a little stuck on this last part, and I asked them to go back into their memories and see what they could come up with. One woman recalled her baby crib. She remembered the quilt and the toys and began to draw this. Another drew a little cottage with yellow curtains and smoke coming out of the chimney. The trees were airy and realistic. Another participant worked on a spring scene. Their work and spirit were so free, the women started to spontaneously sing. I saw this as a great success, not so much in the style of art making, but in the release of feelings.

Session VI

For this session, cups and saucers were set on the table. Later I added cutlery and a teapot. Was this art therapy or an art class? To me, art can be its own therapy. This certainly combined all the elements for having people get involved, in sharing and getting to know one another. Marker pens and colored pencils were the materials chosen— a complete switch from our last session and more controlled. Choosing either medium, they were asked to set up their own still-life. It was challenging to try elliptical shapes and perspective.

At the end of the session, they all stayed for a cup of tea. It wasn't lunch, but even still, having a cup of tea together was a step in the right direction.

Session VII

Today, a small amount of tempura paint was poured into plastic container lids. I brought oranges and peppers from home and sliced them. We used them as stamps and as our inspiration for the day. The group experimented with making prints.

Occasionally, a visitor dropped in. During this session, a daughter and great-grandchild visited. The youngster was thrilled to join the ladies and got right into the materials and the project. This was a wonderful "happening" that could be part of one's master plan, bringing a visitor, planned or spontaneous, after the group has been together for several sessions. (However, one must also take into account the group dynamics, and how the group may feel being "invaded" by newcomers.)

Session VIII

Now that the interaction between the members seemed ongoing, and we had used various art supplies, I was not reticent about asking them to work on a House-tree-person picture (Buck, 1948). (This is a common art therapy diagnostic tool.)The directive proved fruitful, and there was also ample time to share each person's thoughts, memories, and feelings, which added to the information that their artwork provided.

Again at the end of the session, everyone stayed and chatted over a cup of tea. The lunch part still seemed too complicated; however, tea and talk seemed always to be appreciated and a natural way to end the sessions.

Session IX

Since this was so close to a religious holiday (Easter), I wondered if I should even hold the class, thinking that perhaps people would be away visiting relatives or would attend religious services. However, the administration had not said anything about it, so I decided even if only one or two participants arrived, it should go on.

It turned out to be a very important morning. A gentleman resident had died the night before, and some of the people did not know until they arrived at the group. They were all quite upset, and it was evident that their own mortality was at issue here. One of the women remarked that she wanted to "go that way too," speaking of having a peaceful death. There was discussion about eating and drinking habits. One of the women recalled her own father who had always prayed to die in his sleep (and that's what happened). Then another person talked about one of the residents who was quite ill and weak from cancer and chemotherapy treatments. Death and dying was on their minds this Friday morning. I was not sure I could pull them into any activity at all. I questioned myself about whether to encourage them to draw or to just continue with a process group.

My mind was made up as they led the way. Two women said, "Well, what are we doing today? Let's draw eggs." (The Polish woman had already conducted two egg-decorating classes and they were interested in the topic.) In this group, our eggs were going to be drawn on paper (other instructors might want to use actual eggs).

While in the midst of this activity, another woman appeared at the doorway. She was not a participant in the group, but decided to sit and watch. It turned out that she was also upset about the man who had died and needed to be with the others. She was also concerned with yet another resident who had to go back to the hospital but was coming home this very day. This woman was of German heritage. She claimed she could not draw, but then proceeded to execute an elegant and colorful design. One lady suggested it looked like a Faberge egg because it was so jewel-like. As we worked, I reminisced about an Easter from my own youth, a perfectly neutral story, which then started off a flood of memories for the group. The German woman recalled walking in the woods with her parents one cold Easter. She mentioned that they were very poor. During the walk, her father ran ahead now and then. Coincidentally, she would shortly thereafter find a chocolate egg, which she would hand to her mother to put in the basket. When they got home, she asked for her chocolate eggs. There was only one! Her parents continually recycled the one chocolate egg they had for her in the egg hunt. But even worse, her mother had eaten much of it. She said that when she came to America, she felt that that was when her life began. It was the first real freedom she had. She loved to overindulge her children when they were young.

Then the Polish woman had a story to tell. She explained how she would never forget a particular Good Friday during World War II. It was a late Easter that year; she was a young woman, and very religious. It was the custom to visit area churches that day, but this was a highly dangerous activity as the Nazis were stopping people on the main roads. She then recalled further, and told about the parish priest who had dared to make a political statement of sorts by decorating the cross. He was shot. On her way home, people told her to go another way, but this was really the only way possible to reach her home. It was not far from a Jewish ghetto. She saw two children, sick and thin, running for their lives. She witnessed a soldier hurling a grenade at them, which blew them away. At this point in the story, she stopped and cried. There was utter silence in the room.

The German woman then arose to leave the room, perhaps to attend to something, or just for relief. She returned a short time later and said "I am no longer a German. I am an American. Many things happened that I didn't want or like." People get caught in the crossfire of history and these women have seen and experienced things that this spoiled American could not imagine. It was amazing to witness such a powerful exchange, so many years after the event.

Even after this intense period, the women began to relax, talking and coloring their pictures. As I sat with them, I thought of how I almost had not come this morning, which turned out to be one of great importance and need. Just then, the German-born woman, who had finished her lovely egg design, folded the paper to make it into a greeting card. She passed it around the table for all to sign for the friend coming home from the hospital this day. This little act of generosity seemed to bind up the hurtful memories and make for an upbeat closure to a heavy morning. The focus was on life. Everyone took their egg and cross decorations to hang on their doors.

During this group, with their permission, a photo was taken of the entire group with a small story and sent to the newspaper. The director of the apartment complex wanted to promote the facility and introduce the occupants of the building to the community via a photo and article. The participants were asked if they would be willing to be photographed. They welcomed the idea.

The "simple" Easter theme brought up plenty, especially when they were dealing with the death of one friend and the illnesses of some of the other residents, as well as painful memories of their youth. It was humbling and gratifying at the same time to hear the powerful stories these women had to share. They have had profound life experiences and it was amazing to have them open up and release their feelings. I felt entrusted with something very special that day.

Session X

The woman who had received the "welcome home" card last week came to this session. This time, I incorporated some gentle exercises, stretching, and deep breathing into the group, and played some soothing music in the background. I asked the group members to think of some gift they had received and then draw it. One woman drew a country scene with a man and dog walking ahead down the road, another drew a teapot with a smiling face. One had received a beautiful wreath for Mother's Day which she had put on her door, and she drew that. And a flower with a smiling face was drawn by someone else. Each person shared their story of what they had received. Next, I had them trace or draw their hand and put a gift in it for someone at the table. They presented their wishes to each other for health, for an answer to a special prayer, for their families. These simple gestures of kindness to each other were a touching metaphor for the developing gift of friendship and trust they shared.

Session XI

Spring was here and we were almost finished with our 12 sessions. On the way to the group, I grabbed a bunch of daffodils from the garden. In thinking about asking them to draw the flowers, I realized that it was a more complicated project, but thought they were up to the challenge. (I suggest that a variety of flowers be brought in so that they could choose the shapes and colors they preferred. Also, I would suggest to bringing enough flowers to make a small and gracious gift to the participants.)

When they had finished the day's project, I took the opportunity to remind everyone that this was our next-to-last session.

Session XII

In this session, I had them draw something in pencil only. The results were amazing. They were to draw a face and then tell a story about the person. One drew a girl that had been in her class at school who had become a nun, another drew a grandchild. One woman drew a go-go dancer "who really doesn't like doing that." One woman drew her husband. "He doesn't smile much, he is quiet. People sometimes think he is not nice because of that—but he is a good guy."

Finally, we ended with another scribble game. Each person started a picture with some simple mark or line and then passed it on. Then the next person did something to it, until everyone at the table had added something to each picture. When they got their original piece back, they could finish it off and then tell the story. I told them that the others could add to the story, just as they added to the drawing and changed it. It proved to be a creative exercise, lots of fun, and a nice way to end the series at the apartments. It showed me, as it showed them, how the circle of friendship between them had come into being, as they all explored their creativity together.

CONCLUSION

My volunteer work was done when this group ended. I did not continue at the apartments, due to other commitments. But, I am happy to say, the newly formed friendships continued. This was confirmed by the administrator, and through my own observations, when I stopped by occasionally to say hello. People met in the community room and sat outside as the weather improved. However, unfortunately, they never did artwork at the site again.

Overall, I liked the way the 12 sessions worked, both with regards to quantity and quality. It seems that at times of transition, such as moving into an apartment, seniors need a reason, perhaps even an excuse, to get together, try new things, and meet each other. Art therapy groups are perfect for this, as they help by providing a medium about which older adults can discuss, create, and elaborate on. For further recommendations, I would suggest regular, weekly ongoing meetings, which would be beneficial, both in providing an interesting activity, and in helping people process difficult life situations.

REFERENCES

Betensky, M. (1995). *What do you see?* London: Kingsley Publishers.

Buck, J. (1948). The H-T-P Technique: A qualitative and quantitative scoring method. *Journal of Clinical Psychology Monograph, 5,* 1-20.

Butler, R. & Lewis, M. (1977). *Aging and mental growth.* St. Louis, MO: Mosley Publishers.

Dalley , T. (Ed.). (1992). *Art as therapy.* NY: Routledge.

Davidson, J. & Doka, K. (1993). *Living with grief.* Philadelphia, PA: Brunner Mazel.

Fenton J. (2000). Unresolved issues of motherhood for elderly women with SMI. *Journal of the American Art Therapy Association, 17*(1), 24-30.

Fry, P. (1986). *Depression, stress & adaptation in the elderly.* Rockville, MD: Aspen Publishers.

Landgarten, H. (1981). *Clinical art therapy: A comprehensive guide.* NY: Brunner Mazel.

McGoldrick, M., Pearce, J., & Giordano, J. (Eds.). (1982). *Ethnicity and family therapy.* NY: Guilford Press.

Robbins, A. (1987). *The artist as therapist.* NY: Human Science Press.

Schaverian, J. (1992). *The revealing image.* NY: Routledge.

Wald, J. (1986). Fusion of symbol, confusion of boundaries: Percept contamination in Alzheimer's disease patients. *Journal of the American Art Therapy Association, 3* (2), 76.

SECTION III

WORKING WITH INDIVIDUAL OLDER ADULT CLIENTS

Chapter 9

FINDING HER WISDOM: THE CREATIVE JOURNEY OF AN OLDER WOMAN

KATHY MESSMAN

INTRODUCTION

This is the story of a courageous older woman who trusts her internal, imaginal world to inform and guide her end of life experiences. It is also the story of my experiences as her witness, encounters that encouraged me to trust myself while defining my role as an art therapist. Multiple layers of transition and integration occur for client and therapist engaged in the creative process over time. I will offer a view of the therapeutic relationship from the perspective of healing through empathy (Franklin, 1990), imagination (Watkins, 1984), Third Hand services (Kramer, 1986), and parallel process (Malchiodi, 1996). I hope to present this material in the context of a process of aging that Zalman Schachter-Shalomi (1995) describes with great care and respect. "People don't automatically become sages simply by living to a great age. They become wise by undertaking the inner work that leads in stages to expanded consciousness" (p. 15). This leads me to introduce Jen and the two-year journey we shared.

THE CLIENT

Jen was 91 years old when we met and said that it was important that I know that she had never made art. She had recently moved to the assisted living apartments in a large senior community and was

179

very candid about her experience of that move. She admitted resistance to the whole circumstance, which included the use of a motorized wheelchair. I would soon come to know Jen as a quietly thoughtful, reflective, independent woman with great life experiences. She had lost her husband when her children were young and worked diligently to be a successful single parent. Jen had been an accomplished professional, working with young people in the field of human services. In our many conversations over two years I heard Jen describe her life with modest pride, minimal regret, and wonderful humor. In old age, her memories were rich with fondness for her family, many friends, and acquaintances.

Jen experienced chronic pain in her dominant arm, hand, and one leg, causing her to use them less, thus diminishing her physical strength and mobility. Regrettably, medical conditions (a torn rotator cuff in her dominant shoulder, nerve pain originating in her neck that radiated into her arms and hands, an endocrine disorder, minor cardiac disturbances) that had been well-managed in the past were becoming increasingly difficult to treat. Pushing buttons on a tape recorder, turning book pages, or using writing implements (fine motor activities) were limited because of pain in her fingers. Jen consulted with her physicians and family before arriving at the decision to move to an assisted living setting and use a motorized wheelchair. Her ability to use these relationships was one example of her strength and capacity to advocate for herself.

When we first met, Jen stated that although she had dreaded the move to assisted living, she was pleasantly surprised at how much more autonomy she was experiencing as a result of the increased support. The extra help allowed her to save her energy and invest it in activities she still could accomplish. For example, Jen attempted to do a traditional life review using tape recordings and interview techniques but found it disappointing. She felt it was too distanced and impersonal. Jen chose art therapy as a strategy to manage pain while, hopefully, expanding her fine motor functions. It is helpful to know that as well as engaging in one-on-one art therapy, she also became involved in peer counseling and stress reduction/visualization groups at this time. This alerted me to her ability to integrate losses and accept change. As I reflect back, I recognize Jen's courage in acknowledging her current life challenges and to transcend them through imaginal states.

The Setting

The community where she lived is a nonmedical, apartment community. The assisted living apartments are studio size with a common dining room that accommodates 14 residents per floor. There is a resident assistant on each floor who serves meals, does light housekeeping, laundry, offers stand-by assistance for personal care, and dispenses medications as prescribed and monitored by each individual's physician. Residents must be able to manage their bowel and bladder function, get to meals and appointments, and be able to act independently aside from the assistance described above. It is a home environment community. Each apartment is an individual's private home and is treated as such. All of this is located within a larger community of independent senior apartments. Many residents move from "Independent Living" (IL) apartments to "Assisted Living" (AL) apartments, as their needs change.

There is an attitude within the community culture that makes the move to assisted apartments a difficult transition for most residents. It is a move that brings up fears about loss of independent function and eventual death— an avoided, unspoken reality that assaults residents and staff alike. This hidden, pervasive prejudice about AL and what happens "over there" was also part of Jen's struggle. Reclaimed autonomy achieved through the assistance described above was exciting to her. It was also a source of emotional pain because her friends in IL refused to believe her declarations of enhanced independence. Long-standing relationships became distant or dissolved, causing Jen more loss. It was significant that she sought new support and connection in groups and in art therapy.

The Therapist

Until the time I began working with Jen in 1999, I had spent my professional life as a nurse, and more recently, an art therapist in predominantly medical settings. Working in a different professional environment as a new art therapist on the eve of her 50th birthday, recently relocated to Colorado from California, I was experiencing disruptions in my daily life that made me more sensitive to the realities of my clients. Shaken confidence, resistance to aging, funding strength, and finding resources were our common challenges. Annette Shore's thoughtful discussion of the role of the art therapist in a geriatric setting helped me to gain perspective about my issues, while focusing on the developmental needs, strengths, and resources of my clients. I began to see that I was there to serve as a facilitator who would promote the wisdom of these residents as they came to terms with end of life circumstances. "In older age, there exists the unique opportunity for individuals to synthesize an entire lifetime of experience" (1994, p. 173). Jen's courage and strength in meeting new challenges gave testimony to the truth of these words and taught me to appreciate my own stage-related struggles and successes. I have always felt confident about my ability to create a safe therapeutic space for my clients but working in people's apartments left me searching for well-defined boundaries to contain that space. Sezaki and Bloomgarden's discussion of home-based art therapy with older adults, including such considerations as intrusions by family members and others, the use of personal space, and the therapist's personality, was very helpful (2000, pp. 283-290).

Finally, I had to learn to respect Jen's ability to tolerate failure. This meant that I had to look at my own tolerance of painful feelings as being key to my role as her facilitator. Shore states:

> A significant challenge for the art therapist working with elderly clients is avoiding the temptation to take over the creative process for them. Provision of technical support and encouragement facilitates active engagement and struggle. Patients are often directly faced with their disabling conditions and related grief through the very process that is intended to provide resolution. Sometimes feelings of defeat must be accepted because it is a necessary expression in active struggle. The art therapist's ability to tolerate despair while continuing to offer encouragement in facilitating artistic struggle is essential. (1997, p. 173)

Resolution of my feelings of despair and fear has developed with a daily spiritual practice, personal art making, support through supervision, and nurturance of strong relationships with other art therapists.

The approach of my 50th birthday signaled mid-life transition issues that are described by Bridges as a time when there is a mixture of old and new conditions, "full of promise yet lacking meaning" (1980, p. 43). He offers the idea that the young and the old have a sense of place, while those experiencing middle-age "have lost a sense of belonging." I had certainly experienced disruptions in my life previously, but this lack of a sense of belonging felt elemental, that something essential in me was changing. I found myself taking inventory of my values and habits, as though sorting through old possessions. I felt bored, but newly impassioned; somewhat out-of-control, yet I had clarity. In supervision I came to see that Jen was dealing with out of control life circumstances as well, but more so. I watched her build structure for herself through art making and the use of creative imagination, consciously facing and overcoming obstacles.

Also in supervision, I came to recognize a quality of mentorship in Jen's and my relationship, a process of one woman showing another woman her experiences of living/aging. In her article discussing "parallel process," Malchiodi describes how comparable problems experienced by therapist and client parallel each other throughout therapy, and that the therapist's resolution of her difficulties makes her available to objectively see the larger aspects of the client's problems. (1996, pp. 55-56). Moody in *Spiritual Eldering Newsletter* states "Conscious aging . . . invites us to come out of hiding, stop running, and look at our lives in a deeper, [sic] way" (winter-2001, p. 11). Parallel process observation in supervision supported this "conscious aging" process for me. I came to understand the sense of mentorship I felt, and began to recognize Jen as my student and my teacher, as I was her student and her teacher.

The Therapy

The Contract and Goals

Jen's request to begin art therapy was motivated by her interest in managing her chronic pain and improving her daily routines. We set treatment goals together. Pain management through art making, the creation of a personal pain scale, guided imagery and visualization exercises, and the use of her art as a focal object to help recapture experiences of relief were reviewed. The initial intervention was to obtain an art assessment, and based on that information create a treatment plan to meet the goals listed above. The Diagnostic Drawing Series (DDS) (Cohen, 1994) assessment was explained and completed. I found it to be a comprehensive and useful tool for the first session with Jen. In a concentrated period of time, it gave me invaluable information about Jen's ability to use art materials, take risks, access imagination and memory, develop images, and exhibit her limits related to pain and fine motor function difficulties. When the DDS was periodically included in reviews of her artwork over time, her response was like that of a person coming upon an old friend or favored belonging.

We met in my office, but also in her room when circumstance and desire dictated. Eventually, she also expressed a desire to paint between sessions, so we created an accessible space in her apartment.

The Journey and Art Making

Jen's creative journey and art making can be described in three parts: early, middle, and later sessions. The early sessions were marked by playful curiosity, experimentation, discovery, and mastery as she explored materials, tools, and her ability to make art. The use of images, both concrete (photographs used in collage) and imaginal (visualizations) were introduced in this early phase and continued to be integral to Jen's process throughout.

The middle sessions of Jen's journey relate to the period of time when she had gained considerable mastery of the art materials and expressed confidence in her ability to paint, entering a painting in a community exhibit. During this time she was fairly stable medically and was able to apply what she was learning in art therapy and support groups to manage her pain. She seemed to be thoroughly enjoying her accomplishments.

The later sessions reflect a time of increased loss, reorganization, and reflection, for both of us. There was more imaginal exploration with less actual art making by Jen. Her images had become more important to her than her physical condition and, although she was not actively painting as much herself, she was more involved in discussion about her imaginings.

Early Sessions

After Jen's completion of the DDS, I evaluated her strengths related to physical ability and limitations, skill, and style in using art materials, as well as her attitudes and interests in terms of art making. Jen reported that she had never made art in any form but was curious to see what happened. The chalk pastels used for the DDS were hard for her to hold. Small, controlled movements caused severe burning and aching in her hand and arm so her marks were light. Although she liked the results of her drawings she said she found using the chalks difficult and a little frustrating because intense effort produced such a light mark. She experimented with chalk pastels on a moistened surface and with large oil pastels. These mediums were more satisfying to her because the marks were easier to make and showed up with greater intensity. Her interest in bold colors became apparent in these early sessions. After exploring mark-making with these materials, I introduced a collage technique using colored tissue and crepe paper with water, glue, and brushes. Edith Wallace discusses her use of colored tissue paper collage as a tool for working with active imagination (1987, p. 120). I wanted to encourage Jen to use her imagination and attraction to bright colors in creating pictures without having to formally draw. Wallace emphasizes a playful, unselfconscious approach that is free of manipulation. This approach resonated for Jen and became the consistent approach in her process of making art. Wet tissue, crepe and handmade paper collage (Figures 9-1 and 9-2), oil and chalk pastel exploration, acrylic, and watercolor paint applications were approached in a playful let's-see-what-happens-with-this attitude. Winnicott's observations about play as the instrument to being creative and using one's whole personality, "to discover the self," came to mind as I watched Jen's playful process (1971, p. 4).

Thanks to relationships fostered with professionals in the occupational and physical therapy fields, I found ways to adapt drawing and painting tools so that Jen could apply water, glue, or paint with greater ease and comfort. I adapted the brushes with foam tubing to enlarge the grasp and relieve pain caused by fine motor movement in her fingers and hands. She wore gloves at this time but eventually gave them up because pulling them on and off became too painful.

After Jen completed this playful, unselfconscious application she became curious and would begin watching for images to reveal themselves. It was at this time that we became more fully engaged in what Kramer refers to as "Third Hand services" (1986). Kramer explains that art therapists must "command a 'Third Hand,' a hand that helps the creative process along without being intrusive, without distorting meaning or imposing pictorial ideas or preferences alien to the client" (pp. 71-72). That as artists we attain skills and understanding while

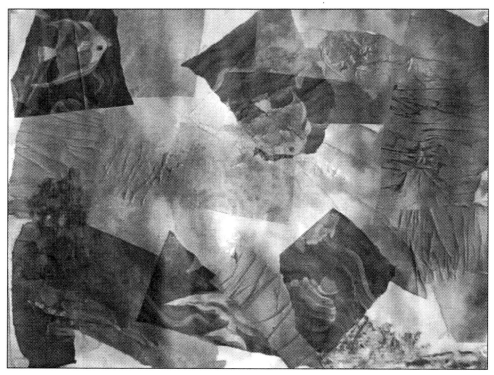

Figure 9-1. Tissue paper collage.

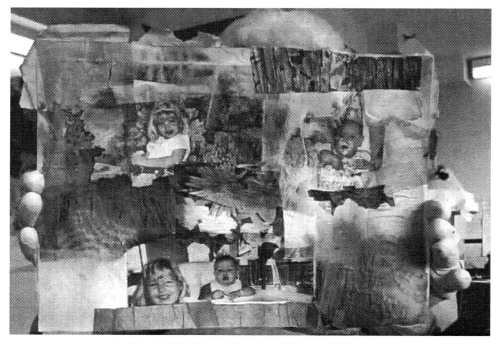

Figure 9-2. Tissue Paper and Photo Collage.

developing our own style, but as art therapists we learn to subordinate our personal style in the service of the client, "to cultivate an area of artistic competence distinct from their own artistic struggles and predicaments, a conflict-free sphere wherein technical skill, pictorial imagination, ingenuity, and capacity to improvise are employed for empathic service to others" (1986, p. 71).

During this time, I began making rough sketches to develop the images Jen found and described to me. This done, she would then begin to develop the images by adding more paint in a purposeful way. She learned to mix color, manipulate materials, and use "accidents" to enhance and develop her images. When something happened that frustrated or disappointed her, she would return to a playful, let's-see-what-happens-if-I-do-this attitude. If she was tired or experiencing pain she would sometimes opt to quit and return to the work later. She was now expressing the desire to paint between our sessions and that led to setting up a space that was ready for her to use at any time she chose, another Third Hand function (Kramer, 1986, p. 72).

Other Third Hand services to Jen were:

- Assessing her skills and capabilities, adapting brushes and drawing implements; experimenting with materials to find the media that was most accessible to her—easiest to manipulate and control without increasing or aggravating pain and fatigue.
- Drawing, cutting, pasting collage elements; constructing while she described composition; sketching the "found" images she described from abstract, random paint applications, her dreams, and her imagery from guided visualization sessions.
- Pacing her efforts to conserve energy and manage pain. This involved observing whether she appeared to be laboring (which in her case might present as a change in skin color) and listening to her voice and breath. Jen would begin to grunt with each exhalation when she was in pain or as she tired. When I observed these symptoms of physical discomfort I would offer her choices to rest, slow down, or stop. Kramer includes in her article a discussion of Theodore Reik's ideas about Third Eye and Third Ear services that closely relate to Third Hand tasks. When old age or illness diminishes the physical capacity to make art, what remains is the ability to make decisions as a way to exercise autonomy. I literally became Jen's muscular strength and physical skill. (1986, p. 71)

Figure 9-3, a collage created from one of Jen's dreams, is an example of an image completed by third-hand intervention through a technique described by Jean Davis (1995) as the "redrawing" of a dream. It is used as a means to move the therapeutic process forward and refers to the process by which a client actually redraws dream imagery (1995, p. 62). In Jen's case I "redrew" the image for her per her direction.

Another aspect of the early period of art making with Jen related to the discussion above concerns the qualities of empathy and aesthetic attitude, an attitude marked by "careful, focused, nonjudgmental absorption in what is being observed" (Franklin, 1990, p. 43). Awareness of a client's physical, emotional, and aesthetic rhythms and offering what is needed is an empathic service. Aesthetic means "artistic" but it also means "visual" and aesthetic attitude for me means that I saw all of Jen, her art making, dreaming, and suffering, and as a result I could empathically respond to her needs. This approach and the empathy I was able to model for Jen allowed her to be a complete beginner who was excited and nonjudgmental while looking for her own unique images and developing them. In periodic reviews, she would rediscover her art and see completed paintings that had merit to her, and even allowed her to exhibit them for others to appreciate. She was not hampered by or concerned about judgment of her work because of my consistent attitude and empathy throughout our work together. My Third Hand service to her in the actions of drawing and sketching demonstrates not only how art making teaches us to feel within ourselves who we are, but also allows us to empathically realize someone else's experience (Franklin, 1990, p. 46).

During the early art-making sessions, I also introduced guided imagery as an imaginal source for Jen. Because she regularly shared her dream experiences and because she was involved in a stress reduction group and was familiar with relaxation techniques and visualization, connecting this practice to our sessions had a natural progression. On days that she was too tired or in too much pain to make art I would lead her in a guided imagery. Afterward she had me draw the images she described (Figure 9-3). This was an incredible experience every time we did it.

She would then direct me to where in her room she wanted it hung so that she could look at it later and "return" to a place that offered comfort and relief. London identifies guided imagery as a restorative

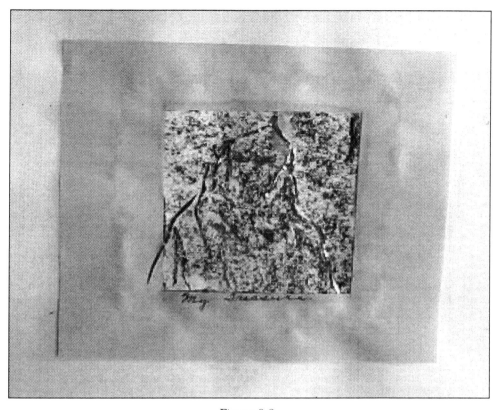

Figure 9-3.

process of creating an inner vision, of physical images of times and places that we travel to through acts of imagination (1989, p. 142). Jen's ability to use this tool to create a restorative environment was primary and constant, and served as a good foundation for her art making.

For example, color images seen in a guided imagery session helped her to create a pain scale that allowed me to evaluate and measure her experience of pain visually. I asked Jen what colors were soothing to her and which might represent pain or discomfort. She then equated representational colors to the numbers 1-10 with one being the least severe intensity and ten the most. Using the pain scale before and after our sessions gave her a concrete measure of what happened when she was involved in the therapeutic process, as well as helping me understand her experience. She also applied the color scale during visualization exercises to sooth her discomfort. By changing the intensity of a color—imaginally decreasing the intensity of a "painful" color or by surrounding herself in a "soothing" color, she changed her experience of pain. Kast speaks to this when she says that our imaginings are a source of hope and our images a reflection of our current condition (1993, pp. 15-16). This is demonstrated in Jen's use of image and color applied to a pain scale.

Figure 9-3 is another example of Jen's art that offered comfort and hope when viewed and reexperienced. Jen's willingness to take risks and keep going was an inspiration to myself and to fellow residents. She participated in a painting group once a week, which was started because she wanted to paint more often and in the company of others. Her progression in art making was affected by changes in her physical condition and my interventions to help her adjust. These interventions were the recurrent catalyst to try new materials, approaches, or tool adaptations. As she began experiencing more pain in her hand we further adapted brushes and thinned acrylic paint with water. This parallel evolution of increasing physical limitations and art-making adjustments led finally to her to the use of watercolors to interpret paintings by other artists such as Georgia O'Keefe and the Impressionists. Sean McNiff's sensitive discussion of risk-taking and how it is essential to the process of finding something fresh and surprising aptly describes what I observed with Jen during our beginning sessions (1992, p. 34).

Middle Sessions

What I consider the middle sessions of Jen's journey relate to the period of time when she was familiar with the materials and exhibited confidence in her ability to make art. She was medically stable for the most part. A therapeutic rhythm had been established; a process of painting, resting, relating experiences with dreams or visualizations, and using the pain scale to measure pain and successfully manage it were all part of the pacing and creating. We continued to meet one-on-one in her room and with a group of four to five other residents who gathered in a common area to paint weekly. Jen was still regularly attending peer counseling and stress reduction groups. She had become confidently assertive in the therapeutic process, asking for help and direction as she needed. I found myself sitting quietly, assisting and facilitating when appropriate, without a lot of dialogue. Rogers describes what I experienced with Jen at this time as a phenomenon called "the full experiencing of an 'affectional relationship'" (1961, pp. 81-82). He states that it occurs in longer work with clients and is not a function of transference/countertransference. When we as therapists are less afraid of our positive (or negative) feelings toward clients there is a shift. Feelings of respect and acceptance for the client change to wonder as we watch the person struggle to become themselves.

Jen's art-making process had a clear sequence of beginning, middle, and completion now. She applied acrylic paint to canvas-paper randomly with a paint knife and then explored the abstract result for images. She would describe what she saw and I would draw a sketch. Then using adapted brushes she applied more paint to develop the images. Her family took her to a framing store to get the finished paintings framed. (Figures 9-4 & 9-5).

Robbins states that finding form in chaos in the creative process is a personal journey (1999, p. 121). The process of taking the chaos of random paint applications and making them into the form of completed paintings is transformational. I believe it empowered Jen to transfer that success to other areas of her life. She would soon experience changes in her physical condition that would require her to move to a new setting. I believe she was better able to embrace and adjust to this change because of her experience of creating form from chaos in art making.

I used my observations of Jen's physical responses during artmaking to teach her to pace herself. Jen had spent her life as a very capable, autonomous individual who had taken pride in her ability to manage well. One of her biggest challenges was to learn this pacing to conserve energy and manage pain. At times in our sessions together I have felt like an official at a sports event, not the focal element of the game but important to its successful completion. I am timekeeper, negotiator, mediator, and resource person. I monitor the time we begin and end, but more important is my role as an observer of her condition as she paints. At first Jen would become so engrossed in the process that she was unaware the she had begun to toil, breathing hard, at times grunting with effort. I would check in with her at these times asking how she felt and pointing out my observation of her condition. She admitted she didn't realize how hard she was working. She would usually choose to rest. I asked her if she wanted me to remind

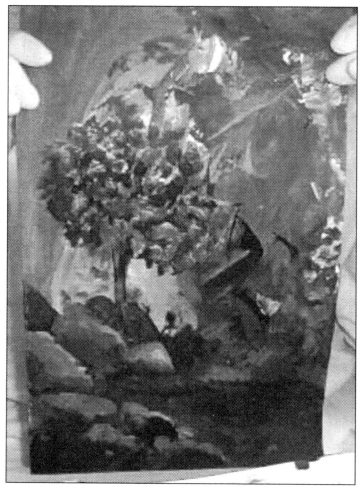

Figure 9-4.

her to stop to rest at shorter intervals and therefore possibly work longer. Her participation in the peer support and stress reduction groups was also enhancing her conscious awareness of her actions and reactions. Although she learned to stop to rest more often she still had difficulty waiting or resting long enough before resuming. Again, I could offer my observations of her physical reactions as information to weigh and decide, thus acting as a mediator and negotiator. As a resource person I would observe her efforts, evaluate how hard it was for her to manipulate a particular medium or tool, offer her choices about her options for accomplishing her objectives, then implement the adjustments so that she could continue.

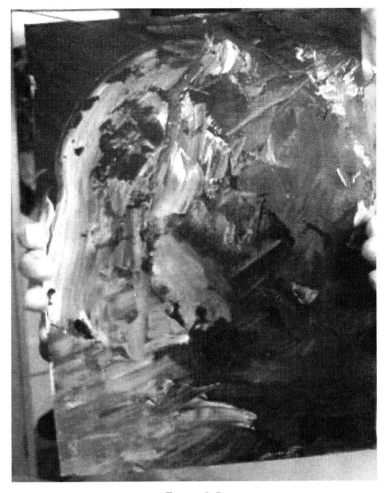

Figure 9-5.

Later Sessions

Art Therapist Michael Franklin states that he sees clients as divine beings and invites the art therapist to orient him/herself to being "open to essence as well as illness, inner as well as outer, known as well as unknown" (1999, p. 6). Jen's physical decline impacted me in a way I had not expected. To remember this the quote above aided me in my experience with Jen; I tried to see all of her, not just the art, or physical symptoms, or the nursing home to which she would soon be moving. To remember to look for the Self that dwells within us all became my work in the later sessions of our journey.

Because of her quietly thoughtful, reflective nature Jen paid close attention and was available to talk about her thoughts and conclusions, as well as her experiences. She became frustrated when her physical condition affected her thinking or her ability to use the tools she had acquired. She was accustomed to using her mind as a valuable instrument and voiced her disgust when it was dulled by illness, dysfunction, medical treatments, and medications. The dilemma of being helped by medical interventions that also encumbered function was a constant in our journey together. We were now moving into an intense time of resolution.

Erikson's discussion of the seventh and eighth stages of development became especially important to me at this time. An urgency I occasionally sensed in Jen had become more intense. Generativity is the urge to leave a legacy, to pass on one's acquired experience to guide the next generation versus letting it languish or stagnate. Successful emotional integration that supports ego integrity leads to acceptance of the responsibility of leadership in old age (1963, pp. 267-269). Overcoming obstacles such as successfully completing her paintings helped produce emotional integration for Jen. Her art became her legacy and the process of art making her declaration of leadership. One day, Jen verbalized her frustration about people wanting her to play trivia games because she knew the answers, but not expressing interest in her paintings which were what was important to her; "They are interested in the trivia I know, how many answers I can get right, and they don't look at or ask about the art I make."

I mentioned earlier that I had strong reactions to Jen's changing condition and this brings me to a discussion of how the feelings of the therapist affect the therapeutic alliance. My feelings included the cumulative losses I had been experiencing prior to her move, the many other residents who had moved or died or were losing function. Robbins addresses my experience in his comments about countertransference and empathic responsiveness.

As therapists we are trapped by the disorganization of our surroundings. Tremendous energy and affects seem to invade our very being. The primitive nature of these powerful forces demands holding and boundaries, as well as the ability to digest the affects carried by all of this energy. (Robbins, 1999, pp. 124-125)

He states that empathic relatedness and countertransference issues cannot be separated. They are part of the mix; my emotional issues stemming from my past experiences, distant and recent, intruded on my empathic availability. Our sessions had become less regular due to Jen's hospitalizations. I found myself avoiding visits, not knowing what to say or offer. Feelings of sadness and helplessness at Jen's worsening condition along with the uncertainty about whether her ability and devotion to art making would be lost, became too great for me. I was unable to maintain the "state of free-floating attention" (Robbins, 1989, p. 17, p. 114) necessary to the therapeutic alliance.

My struggle with my own mid-life transition and in relationships with my aging mother and dead grandmother were brought into play, both informing my work with Jen as well as having the potential to interfere with my effectiveness. I brought these personal issues to supervision as the parallel process work I described previously (Malchiodi, 1996). Thanks to the established routine and structure of supervision, when my difficulty with Jen's increasing frailty and her move arose, I, too, was being held in an established empathic relationship. I, like Jen, had a therapeutic container to hold me as I navigated through feelings brought about by more change, perceived loss, and an uncertain future.

During the period of her move, and for two months afterwards, I did not visit Jen. My fears of her dying, of not being able to help her, of crying in front of her, of her fear/tears, and of my own dependency and death were dealt with in supervision. As a result, I was prepared to hold a therapeutic space when I did reestablish regular sessions with her; she spoke about feeling alone, missing her old home, crying during the night and not knowing why except that she felt so alone, and of not wanting to burden her family. We spoke about depression at these times. She was open to discussion about her feelings and didn't believe that she was feeling anything abnormal or unhealthy. "These feelings aren't comfortable and they don't make much sense but I seem to need to feel them. . . . I would say if I was worried about them. . . . I just feel them and then they pass." We reviewed all of her artwork and visualizations at that time. The review seemed to reassure her. The artwork and her imagery seemed to bring her to her deepest self. "At times like this the ego shrinks and the realm of the self expands and is fostered" (Franklin, 2000, 2001, notes from supervision). Both Jen and I were experiencing an expansion of the

Self, looking within. Letting go of old, defensive ego structures to find strength and resolution in current circumstances. Making sense out of conditions through reflection and internal information, from intuitive sources.

Watkins speaks about our "imaginal egos" as being a great source of insight about the Self. We become a part of the imaginal, moved by it, finding it is a familiar land that feels like home, while what is happening outside of us feels foreign (1984, p. 117-118). "We confuse 'something sick with something wrong' (Hillman, as cited in Watkins, 1984, p. 124). In the material daily world this is so. But it need not be so in the imagination—indeed, it does not seem to be so when we allow ourselves further access to these visions" (Watkins, 1984, p. 123). These insights helped me in our discussions of her feelings of loneliness and depression. When Jen's physical symptoms dulled her senses, she appeared slowed down. She would struggle a little to regain clarity and focus, but was really thriving due to her imaginal world. She expressed more interest and curiosity about her images than about her latest medical evaluation.

Symbols, Pacing, and Empathy

I am not prepared to discuss Jen's images because she did not fully discuss them. I have many ideas about how they might represent her Self, her process, and have had the experience of watching her with her images, knowing that she knows their meaning. She takes them at face value and trusts them. I could go into a long explanation about the literature and what some of her symbols might represent but that does not feel right. That she has great affection and esteem for her imagery, in her artwork as well as her visualizations, is enough for me. At the time of this writing we are still meeting weekly and if an appropriate opportunity arises I would like to invite her to explore a dialogue with her images.

An experience related to her use of imagery that she has shared and I have observed is when she has occasionally looked at one of her animals and commented, "I wonder what it knows?" or when asked about a monk in one of her paintings she matter-of-factly said, "He's me."

Jen has a style of "stopping" in a guided imagery and does not hear the "story" beyond that point until the moment when I invite her back.

One example of this is when she did not find a gift left for her on a bench (part of the narration) because she was attracted to two ducks on a lake (her personal imagery and imagining) down and across a wide expanse of green lawn. When reviewing her guided imagery experiences she consistently reported this point of personal engagement, what I call "stopping." The stopping point was always the focal point in the guided imagery and is what she wanted to speak about or have me draw. Hers was a relaxed attention to and curious observation of something she engaged on the journey. She is a woman of few words who trusts her internal process and imagery. This ability to stop and wait in ambiguity is something she does naturally, with an accepting attitude. It is one of her greatest strengths. Yet when she is painting she relies on me to pace her and show her how to conserve energy. My observation is that she knows how to wait in most things even when frustrated, except when she is physically immersed in the creative process. Then she needed external pacing (a Third Hand service cited earlier). Her rhythm leading mine, her pacing leading mine, is another example of the function of empathy. I "see" her, "hear" her, I am listening on all levels—physical, creative, spiritual. I believe this is why I am able to draw her images so accurately, act as her Third Hand when she paints and I support, and when I narrate and she sculpts her own internal imagery. In the act of pacing, I am like a narrator who is tracking Jen's inner and outer experiences. All of this feels like mentorship and has become the foundation for mapping my work with elders.

One important aspect of our work was the periodic review of Jen's artwork—the body of work viewed together. Her acceptance of her accomplishments was verbalized at these times, although for the most part, the symbolism was not discussed. "I like that more each time I see it. . . . It really is pretty good. . . . I thought it wasn't very good but now I see that I really did do a good job on it. . . . I'd like to work on that some more, finish it." Her expression of affection for and attachment to her art as well as her report of her family's attraction to her artwork was a source of pride. She also was clear about keeping the art in her room and visible or easily accessible, saying, "I'll keep them until I'm finished with them. I'm not ready to let them go . . . I'm not ready yet." Leaving a legacy for her family was being fulfilled for her, the urge for generativity satisfied.

Having weathered a painful transition together, the later sessions have been rich with new traditions. We visit socially, Jen asking for news of her old friends, and me asking about family and current events in her life. Then we engage in art making.

CONCLUSION

Kerr discusses the reexamination of conventional views of aging as a relevant social issue to be addressed by art therapists, stating that art therapy with elders is an acknowledgement of their inner life as being "as viable and salient as earlier transitional stages such as adolescence and mid-life" (1999, p. 38). Experiencing my own mid-life transition while guiding Jen's creative journey in older age led me to be curious, to reevaluate my ideas about myself, art making, being a therapist and caregiver. McNiff's statement, "I learned by watching, and the patients taught me the simple lessons of painting in a natural style" (1992, p. 33), took on a much more powerful meaning for me. I have come to realize that as I have watched Jen, I have also been learning the simple lessons of life in a "natural style," letting her show me the wisdom while she was finding it. I have had to slow down, to be at her pace, and have learned incredible lessons in doing so. I realize that she has been pacing me.

I personally experience art as a spiritual occupation in which I become absorbed and transformed; I know this from my insides. As I have participated with Jen on her journey, I have experienced someone else's spiritual journey and have received a deep sense of knowing, from the outside. Jen has developed the images in her paintings and finds them in other settings in her environment, the figures she perceives in a rock wall outside her room. I am coming to understand that "the more intense our involvement with our images becomes, the greater their significance to us will be, and the more likely it is that we may be able to have experiences comparable to those the mystics had" (Kast, 1993, p. 17). This supports my belief that the last period of life is a time of wisdom and hope where we have the awesome opportunity to receive incredible creative vitality and to use it to explore and offer a legacy. When I told Jen about this chapter and asked her whether she wanted to participate, she was very definite in her desire to have it written. It is a container for the work we have done and fulfills the need to pass on her experience and wisdom, her legacy.

Writing it has reconfirmed for me that art therapy is the container to hold the compassion I feel for our elders as they step into their power as our sages.

Reflecting on what the creative process has given Jen, I find the synonyms for the word "creativity" informative. Originality, imagination, inspiration, ingenuity, inventiveness, resourcefulness, and vision are all listed, and as I think about each word as it relates to Jen's journey I find resonance. Physical limitations, loss of strength and vitality, diminished concentration, discomfort, failure, and frustration were constant companions on this journey, yet the act of creating sustained and expanded Jen's world. As her external, physical world became more restrictive, her imaginal world grew, giving her internal resources to nourish her and enrich her life. Her family has watched in awe and has been enriched as well. I have a sense of gratitude that only tears express.

REFERENCES

Bridges, W. (1980). *Transitions: Making sense of life's changes.* New York: Addison-Wesley.

Cohen, B. M., Mills, A., & Kijak, A. K. (1994). An introduction to the diagnostic drawing series: A standardized tool for diagnostic and clinical use. *Art Therapy: Journal of the American Art Therapy Association, 11*(2), 105-110.

Davis, J. (1995). Processing dream images within the context of art therapy as an approach to personality integration. *Pratt Institute Creative Arts Therapy Review, 16,* 57-63.

Erikson, E. (1963). *Childhood and society.* New York: W.W. Norton.

Franklin, M. (1990). The esthetic attitude and empathy: A point of convergence. *American Journal of Art Therapy, 29,* 42-46.

Franklin, M. (1999). Becoming a student of oneself: Activating the witness in meditation, art, and super-vision. *American Journal of Art Therapy, 38,* 2-13.

Franklin, M. (2000). Notes from supervision.

Kast, V. (1993). *Imagination as space of freedom: Dialogue between the ego and the unconscious.* (A. Hollo, Trans.). New York: Fromm International.

Kerr, C. C. (1999). The psychosocial significance of creativity in the elderly. *Art Therapy: Journal of the American Art therapy Association, 16*(1), 37-41.

Kramer, E. (1986). The art therapist's third hand: Reflections on art, art therapy, and society at large. *American Journal of Art Therapy, 24,* 71-86.

London, P. (1989) To the land of peace and well-being: Guided imagery. In *No more secondhand art: Awakening the artist within.* Boston: Shambhala.

Malchiodi, C. A., & Riley, S. (1996). *Supervision and related issues: A handbook for professionals.* Chicago: Magnolia Street Publishers.

McNiff, S. (1992). *Art as medicine: Creating a therapy of imagination.* Boston, MA: Shambahala.

Moody, H. R. (Winter 2001). Conscious aging festival planned. *Spiritual Eldering Newsletter, 5*(1), 1, 11-12.

Robbins, A. (1989). *The psychoaesthetic experience: An approach to depth-oriented treatment.* New
     York: Hunan Sciences Press.

Robbins, A. (1999). Chaos and form. *Art Therapy: Journal of American Art Therapy Association,
     16*(3), 121-125.

Rogers, C. R. (1961). *On becoming a person: A therapist's view of psychotherapy.* Boston: Houghton
     Mifflin.

Schachter-Shalomi, Z., & Miller, R. S. (1995). *From aging to saging.* New York: Warner Books.

Sezaki, S. & Bloomgarden, J. (2000). Home-based art therapy for older adults. *Art Therapy:
     Journal of the American Art Therapy Association, 17*(4), 283-290.

Shore, A. (1997). Promoting wisdom: The role of art therapy in geriatric settings. *Art Therapy:
     Journal of the American Art Therapy Association, 14*(3), 172-177.

Wallace, E. (1987). Healing through the visual arts – a Jungian approach. In J.A. Rubin (Ed.),
     Approaches to Art Therapy: Theory and Technique (pp. 114-133). New York: Brunner/Mazel.

Watkins, M. (1984). *Waking Dreams.* Woodstock, Connecticut: Spring Publications.

Winnicott, D. W. (1971). *Playing and Reality.* New York: Tavistock/ Routledge.

Chapter 10

ART THERAPY AND ALZHEIMER'S DISEASE: MY MOTHER'S ART

Linda Lee Goldman

A SOUL LOOKING OUT[1]
Color surrounds her
Blending of nature
The depth of a spirit
The eye of a storm
A whirlpool
Swirling autumn leaves
Eyes of sadness
A bruise
Mirage
Looking into space
Cock-eyed world
Farmland, distant fields
A soul looking out

INTRODUCTION

This chapter represents a 15–year journey that I have personally experienced with my mother and her struggle with Alzheimer's Disease. I have included samples of her art before and after the onset of the disease.

As part of the disease process, the Alzheimer's patient goes through various stages of mental and physical diminishment, which require dif-

---

1. Poem constructed from words spoken by group members upon viewing the image in Figure 10.1 created by my mother.

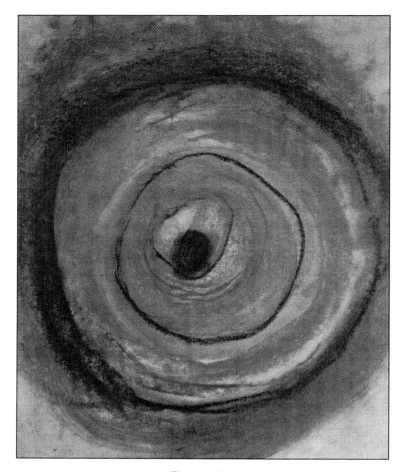

Figure 10-1.

ferent facilities, different types of care, and different types of care-givers. During each stage of her disease and at each facility where she resided, I witnessed a glaring lack of appropriate programming for patients with her problem. This stimulated me to establish art therapy programs for Alzheimer's patients, which I have described in this chapter.

Mom is now curled up in a near fetal position, her hands, held tightly over her chest, seem to guard her. One is open, the other is a closed fist. I open up her hand and wash it with warm water and then give her something soft to hold on to. She cannot speak. At this very late stage of Alzheimer's disease, when I visit, when I speak or touch her, her expression subtly shifts from glazed and distant to soft and connected.

MY MOTHER ESTHER'S HISTORY

Esther, my mother, was born in a small Wisconsin town. Her parents owned a fruit and vegetable business selling their products from a horse-drawn wagon. Mom met her husband, my father, at age 14 and they married when she was 19. Esther was a kind, goodhearted woman and was extremely social and loved by all. She was a loving wife and a nurturing, caring mother.

While I was growing up, my mother would often say to me, "I wish I could paint that sunset," or, "I wish I could paint that sunrise," but in her young adulthood she had never made art. Her life was centered around her family, raising her children, being with her friends and doing community work. She was known for her good cooking, especially her baking. The neighborhood children called her "the cookie lady." They would frequently stop by her house for treats. Although she often admired art, it was not something she thought about creating for herself. She was busy with child-rearing, family life, socializing, and especially taking care of her husband.

However, in mid-life she began to take painting lessons for her own enjoyment. She continued taking these classes for several years. Her art was passionate, full of momentum and color. She painted those things that she loved: her husband golfing, her cocker spaniel, children, and nature scenes. Then at age 60, she took on a full-time job as a receptionist, learned to operate a computer, then and stopped making art.

My mother was in love with life. She was resilient to the multitude of shifts, changes, and surprises that life brought to her. She was a receptionist at a local suburban hospital for 13 years, until her memory problems made continuing there impossible. Unaware of the reason for her dismissal, she was devastated. Later, when my parents could no longer manage their home of 40 years, I helped them move to a retirement community.

LIFE IN THE RETIREMENT COMMUNITY

Shortly after my parents moved to the retirement community, I developed an Expressive Arts Program there. My mother was a mem-

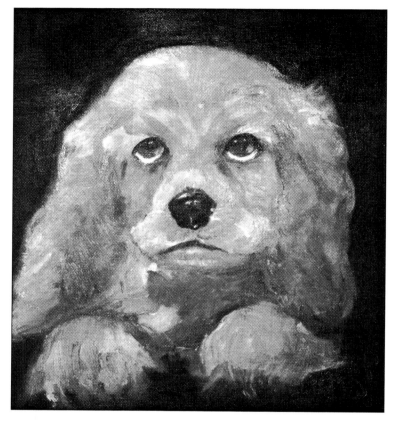

Figure 10-2. Dog painted before Alzheimer's.

ber of this group and looked forward, as did other residents, to our weekly meetings. Initially, she was able to navigate to the art room without help. As her deterioration progressed, she lost that ability and needed a full-time caretaker. Towards the end of her stay at the retirement community, she was unable to hold on to a thought even momentarily. This issue became evident in her daily life. For example, my mom had always had dark, beautiful, well-arched eyebrows, always well-accented with each brow neatly lined. One day, I picked her up at the retirement community to attend her dear friend's funeral. On this occasion, she had substituted lipstick instead of eyeliner. Also, most of the time, even though her husband might be sitting right next to her, she would question with great concern where he was. Eventually, it was decided that a move into an Alzheimer's facility was appropriate.

Even after her move to the facility, we continued to make art together. This art making continued until she physically could not manipulate a brush or mentally focus on any object, or even recognize a dog, her favorite animal. While she was able to make art, she was able to sublimate her free flowing anxiety and fear into a form. At one point, while doing a tracing of her hand, she held that hand out to me and questioned, "Where did I go wrong? Why is God punishing me?" (See Figure 10-3.)

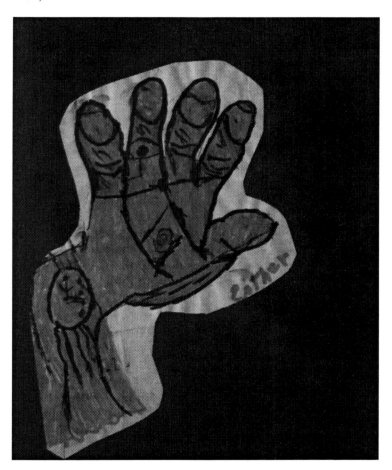

Figure 10-3. Why is God punishing me?

ALZHEIMER'S DISEASE

Alzheimer's Disease and Related Disorders: An Overview

Dementia is the loss of mental function in two or more areas such as language, memory, visual and spatial abilities, or judgment severe enough to interfere with daily life. Dementia itself is not a disease but a broader set of symptoms that accompanies certain diseases or physical conditions. Well-known diseases that cause dementia include Alzheimer's disease, multi-infarct dementia, Parkinson's disease, Creutzfeldt-Jakob disease, Pick's disease, and Lewy body dementia. . . . Individuals experiencing dementia-like symptoms should undergo diagnostic testing as soon as possible. An early and accurate diagnosis helps to identify reversible conditions, gives patients a greater chance of benefiting from existing treatments, and allows them and their families more time to plan for the future.

Alzheimer's disease (AD) is the most common of dementia, affecting as many as four million Americans. AD is a degenerative disease that attacks the brain, begins gradually, and progresses at a variable rate. AD results in impaired memory, thinking, and behavior and can last from three to 20 years from the time of onset of symptoms. Warning signs of AD are memory loss that affects job/home skills, difficulty performing familiar tasks, problems finding the right words, disorientation as to time and place, poor or decreased judgment, difficulty with learning and abstract thinking, placing things in inappropriate places, changes in mood and personality, and marked loss of initiative. In the last stage of AD, patients are unable to take care of themselves (Alzheimer's Disease and Related Dementias Fact Sheet, 1999).

THE STAGES OF ALZHEIMER'S DISEASE

An Alzheimer's patient goes through various stages, and impairments develop at unpredictable rates with differing severity. Health care professionals generally categorize the disease into early, middle, and late stages.

Hellen (1992), in her book *Alzheimer's Disease Activity Focused Care*, outlines the stages of the disease as follows. The early stage/mildly impaired is typically one to three years in duration. This stage is characterized by memory loss and increasing difficulty in the more complicated brain functions. Driving a car or managing finances may become too difficult. Socially, the person is more comfortable in smaller groups and with well-known family and friends. Already established activities are still enjoyed, however learning new information or new activities becomes impossible.

The middle stage/moderately impaired is five to seven years in duration, but can be much longer. This stage is characterized by written and spoken language difficulties; it is common to ask questions repeatedly. Finding the right words or following a conversation becomes difficult. Delusions or paranoid behavior are not uncommon during this stage. This is partly because the person has reduced or absent short term memory. Misplacing objects under these circumstances easily leads to agitation. Patients wandering, pacing, and rummaging through personal belongings is common. Personal hygiene and clothing selection also becomes difficult.

The late stage/severely impaired is two to three years in duration, but can be much longer, often depending upon the quality of nursing care. This stage is characterized by the inability to remember most things or to care for one's own basic needs. Major language difficulties are present and the names of immediate family are forgotten. The person may recognize his/her loved one, but might not be able to use or remember his or her name. Mobility becomes unsteady or impossible, as muscles and joints become rigid. However, even in this last stage, the individual responds to the emotions of anger, happiness, and love. Although the words of the caregivers may not be understood, communication of feelings by expression, touch, and body language is possible (Hellen, 112, pp. 141-143).

WATCHING ONE'S PARENTS AGE

Alzheimer's is a humiliating, devastating experience that strips the individual of all that he/she has known, worked for, and striven for. In some sense, it is of greater magnitude than physical death, for it is a death of a human's spirit, his/her very soul. As children and young adults, our parents seem young and vibrant to us. They are our ideal and our hope. When we are in our mid-life, our parents may begin to fail, physically and mentally. They may have difficulty seeing, hearing, or digesting their food. Most piercingly devastating is that their memories start to fail. They may not seem to know us or remember even their own lives and seem to have lost their sense of self.

One day, while visiting my mother in her retirement community, I asked her, "How are you today, Mom?" "How well can you be when you don't know where you are?" she replied.

I witnessed her slow decline. I watched her life narrow and her options become limited. Some of these limitations were secondary to the disease process and some were because of limitations of our health care system, specifically with respect to care given patients with Alzheimer's disease.

I found that many nursing facilities do not nurture or feed the souls of their residents. Although some residents are able to manage well and accept their limitations, those who cannot rally for themselves and have no one to care for them rely on the varying capabilities of the staff in these facilities.

> Gerontological literature consistently stresses the fact that we as a society have no guiding vision or image of meaningfulness or purpose regarding growing old. . . . The lack of vision in the value of aging manifests itself in geriatric services and programs that are bereft of meaning. Programming has its focus keeping people busy and arranging opportunities for socializing. Socializing is not bad, in and of itself, but when it consists of playing childish games, watching television, and making prefabricated crafts, it is without depth or integrity. The arts can be of immense service in balancing this situation by attending to the question of meaning from a spiritual perspective. For me, this quest for meaning in art and art making has found form in the principles and practices of shamanism (Rugh, 2001, p. 167).

I constantly struggled with the task of how I could preserve the integrity, the experiences that enlivened the spirit of my mother as well as that of other Alzheimer's patients who lacked the physical and emotional capabilities to help themselves? I felt like a cheerleader holding on tight to my mother's history—my own history.

Robert Galatzer-Levy and Bertram Cohler (1993), in their book *The Essential Other*, discuss a psychoanalytic investigation of the older adult. "The self develops across the whole course of life through relations with others. . . . The essential other is our experience of other people, and entities in the environment, that supports the sense of a coherent and vigorous self and its development" (p. 3). "Others" needed for development are not only people, but also communities, institutions, ideas, and stories. The authors explore how we maintain the sense of personal integrity in our adult years (Galatzer-Levy & Cohler, p. 3).

I believe, as an art therapist, that art making can and does serve and substitute for an "essential other." Those who are rich with "essential others" have the capacity to thrive more easily than those who do not. Art can be an enlivening "essential other" for the older adult. The art-making experience may be especially significant to those who are experiencing the early and middle stages of Alzheimer's disease. The art experience may serve as solace, when established essential others can no longer serve that purpose. Learning to accept another's reality and being able to work with that reality, even when it becomes considerably different from ours, is the work of intimacy—heart work. Walking in another's shoes with understanding and empathy while still connected to our own experience and reality is the work of compassion. Helping our parents as they age and die calls for this understanding and compassion and we can find ourselves transformed in the process (Hardin, 1992, p. 205).

OUR JOURNEY THROUGH ART

Fifteen years ago, I expressed to several friends my concern about my mother's memory loss. Upon hearing this, one said, "Do you think your mother has Alzheimer's disease?" Initially, I angrily rejected that concept as impossible; however, I later realized that, indeed, my mother was in the early stages of the disease. Now, in the late stages, she is unable to speak, walk, or move her arms or legs and is apparently unaware of her surroundings.

I sit with her in her bedroom. We are surrounded by the paintings that she did before the onset of Alzheimer's disease. I often give her something soft, such as a beanbag, or stuffed toy animal to squeeze. Sometimes I play piano for her or leave the radio on playing classical music for her to hear. I often write in my daily journal about those visits with her. It is nourishing and connecting for me to imagine what I think, wish, or hope she is experiencing and how I might soothe her. I hold her, stroke her, kiss her on the forehead and tell her stories.

The following is a poetic reflection that I wrote in spring of 2003.

> When I look into her eyes
> What do they say?
> I see you
> I know you
> Seeing you I know I exist
> Seeing you is home, familiar
> Seeing you I love again.
> I hear you
> I know your voice
> I smile inside and out
> Thank you for not forgetting who I am
> When I don't know who or what or where or how I am.
> Thank you for really talking to me when I can no longer speak.
> Thank you for love
> You give it to me
> And I feel it in my heart
> And know I exist
> Thank you love.

I cannot relate at all to her now, or figure out what she is experiencing. Only her eyes, so bright and alive and telling, give me an indication that all of her is not gone. As my mother's functional level deteriorated, it was necessary to move her to various facilities appropriate to those levels. When I would visit her at various placements, I would always bring a watercolor set with large brushes or chalks. During these visits, we would routinely sit and make art. Occasionally, other residents would join us in our art-making activity. When they painted with us, I observed their transition from resigned boredom and sleepiness to interest and excitement.

Art Making: Our Creative Process

It is important to nurture the innate creativity we all possess. Art making in itself is a form of alchemy, making something out of raw materials. ". . . Our sensations are the doorway to understand one another. A doorway allows one to move from one place to another. Sensations are the doorway to art expression, and art may very well be the ultimate form of communication because it makes visible the invisible" (Seiden, 2001, p. 15). Art making is a way of attaching meaning to, and putting into symbolic form, our experiences. As one's emotional and cognitive reality changes, the images one creates also change.

I have worked with a variety of aging adults—from those with normal aging-related issues, to those with extreme deterioration due to Alzheimer's disease. Through making art with my mother and other Alzheimer's patients, I witnessed the ability of how those with limited cognitive capabilities are nonetheless able to express their emotional and cognitive realities through this process. Her art and that of the others in her group validated this process for me, as an imperative part of interactive experiences for those suffering with the devastating impact of this disease.

I was frustrated by my perception of the lack of appropriate activities for the Alzheimer's population, within the health care system. This frustration stimulated me to create art-making programs at the various facilities in which my mother resided. It seemed to be much easier for me to facilitate an art-making group with her and her fellow residents, than to visit with my mother, only to watch her and others sit in a group, sometimes dozing off, while a staff member tried to lead them in activities to which they could not relate. I would often observe bored workers fall asleep themselves when it was their turn to lead an activity. Voicing this frustration to the various administrations of these facilities enabled me to officially create these art therapy groups.

My Mother's Art: The Early Stage

When I first began working with my mother, I would actually draw on the images that she was creating. Early in my art therapy training, I had learned never to do this. Despite my training, this was my attempt to block, resist, and deny the flood of feelings that would emerge when I began to realize that she was losing control and organization of her images. I also felt frustrated about not being able to control her disease-related degeneration. I wanted her to stay focused and to see the difference between background and foreground. She couldn't. When I drew on her work, she would typically obliterate my lines. It became a battle of the chalks. Many of her early images contain my obliterated structure lines. My efforts were actually annoying to her. It took me a long time not to try to hold her form together with my lines.

In the early stages of her disease, all she really needed was a piece of paper and art materials. She was quite able to enjoy her art-making process without my well-meaning, but misguided, help. During this stage, my mother was highly motivated, enjoyed the process, and was receptive to the group member's comments about her artwork. She would also comment on other group member's art. (See Figure 10-4.)

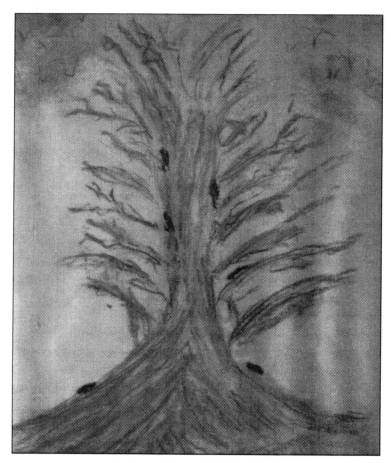

Figure 10-4. "I miss my home and trees and squirrels": Early stage.

MY MOTHER'S ART: THE MIDDLE STAGE

Having given up the battle of the chalk, now I aided her by guiding her spontaneity and witnessing her new emerging style. The progression of her disease was mirrored by her decreasing capacity to create and hold onto form as she had done in the past. Her warmth of color and rhythmic movements, however, continued. Even as she reached ever-lowering levels of organization, and her ability to connect her thoughts decreased, her art making continued to be soothing and delighting for her. In the earlier stages, her art appeared almost cancerous, macabre, angry, sad, and dark. This may have reflected her struggle with the shift in functioning and the fear that accompanied cognitive changes. During the beginning of the middle stage, her artwork changed and became colorful and cheerful. When the internal shift was complete, her images shifted from a variety of shapes and forms to only circular motions.

I had no intention in creating a "therapeutic" art therapy relationship with my mother. However, being part of her art-making process also assisted me to accept her degeneration. Through viewing her images, I could empathize more with her struggle. Art making also kept my mother interested and stimulated, and gave me a focus when visiting with her.

My development of the art groups was a transitional time for me to accept, learn, and assist her. The art-making process was anchoring and focusing for her. Art was a way to be with her in a more meaningful and enjoyable way. As a daughter with a mother struggling with Alzheimer's disease, making art together became a natural way to be with her. I continued to make art with my mother until her condition made that activity impossible. Music and touch, my presence and a smile, now, are the only avenues of contact.

My Personal Art

Art making allows me the time to absorb a feeling and an awesome experience deeply, and to honor its unique character. This can happen to anyone who embraces the playfulness as well as the seriousness of an art-making experience. It's enjoyable, it can be hard work, but most of all, it can release and relieve emotions that one cannot express in other ways.

During the fall, I usually have the need to paint with yellow and orange as a way of honoring the seemingly spiritual warmth that filters through the golden forest cathedral trees into me. Winter light, after trees are bare and the snow has fallen, casts shadows of blue and mauve across the diamond-like snow. With paintbrush in hand, it becomes imperative that I use the intensity I feel towards life, expressing that intensity in an image, allowing it to emerge through symbolic expression in lines, shapes, colors, dimension, and rhythm. I attempt to capture a moment in time. I try to assist those I work with to do the same.

Interestingly, as my mother's art lost structure and form, I began to experience a new rigidity in my own artwork. For over 30 years, I have studied and painted the human figure, especially as portraiture. Painting the figure was a way for me to study the human condition. It also enabled me to develop my own intra-psychic development. As my mother's condition steadily deteriorated, I found myself painting even more realistically. In this way I sublimated my wish to control her disease. I did a portrait of my father that was probably the most realistic portrait I have ever done. This pastel marked the end of my portrait period. Within the structure lines this portrait reflected his sadness as well as my own.

With the dramatic shift in my family structure and my increasing role in the personal care of aging parents, I no longer found portraiture nourishing. I discovered new personal restoration through the delightful capabilities inherent in watercolors. Hungrily, I painted images from nature. I found this new medium and subject matter soothing and curative. The magic of watercolor spontaneously released pleasure and soothed me during this difficult life passage.

This release is what I want for the Alzheimer's residents to experience, on whatever level they are capable of doing so.

ART THERAPY WITH PERSONS WITH ALZHEIMER'S

Benefits of An Art Therapy Program

With the proper in-service training from an expressive therapist, staff at a nursing facility (including nurses, therapists, and volunteers) may be trained to facilitate an atmosphere of creative possibilities for the residents.

There are many opportunities for stimulating and successful art experiences for patients with limited capabilities. Each phase of Alzheimer's disease brings new limitations as well as possibilities. The art therapist must try to make these limitations and difficulties work for the client, not against them. Safety, of course, is paramount. If, for example, patients are unable to use specific materials because they might eat them, edible materials such as pudding, food-coloring, or dark colors of powdered drink mixes can be substituted as a medium. The following summarizes some of the qualities inherent in making art with Alzheimer's patients.

Stimulates Spontaneity

Although Alzheimer's disease restricts communicative abilities, it does not eliminate expression until the very late stages. An expressive therapist can guide the Alzheimer's patient into spontaneity with materials compatible with their individual limitations.

Engages Playfulness

Boredom and complacency can be transformed into stimulation and pleasure not only through participation but also through observation. Thus, the staff indirectly benefits as well.

Externalizes the Internal

We do not know how an individual perceives the world around them as the disease progresses. The process of making art assists patients to externalize the internal, to express what they cannot say and to anchor themselves. When we view their images we are allowed a glimpse of their inner experience. Art therapy groups open up new understandings of Alzheimer's patients while giving us insight into their individual essences.

Creates Organization

Art expression offers the Alzheimer's patient a way to organize that which seems unorganizable to the observer. It is important to allow the patient to experiment freely with appropriate materials so as not to undermine possibilities. The process of making art becomes an avenue of stimulation and communication. The power of art can allow the individual with Alzheimer's to find a place where their usually pent-up emotions can flow and take form.

Evokes Muscle Memory

Muscle memory is engaged by the movement of a paintbrush, dabbing with a sponge, or movement with drawing materials as the patient creates images and designs. Muscle memory assists individuals to organize their world on their own terms. Art therapy can open up wonderful new worlds.

Activates the Senses

Activation of the senses can be a first step away from the Alzheimer's patient's imprisonment within the solitary confinement of the self. Using art materials can develop and give "play" to all of the natural senses.

Evokes Different Emotions and Memories

Feelings of pleasure may be stimulated with clay work. Aggression may be relieved by pounding nails and woodworking. Anxiety may be soothed by painting. Utilization of all five of the senses must be incorporated in the therapeutic settings.

Gives Individuals a Sense of Control

Through manipulation of materials, choosing colors, and all the other choices inherent in art making, those with limited resources may feel a sense of control as well as become relaxed and soothed. This is especially important at the time of their lives when everything else seems out of control or controlled by someone else.

Allows Safe Self-Expression and Freedom

Group members can talk, sing, laugh, and cry as well as move freely inside the boundaries of a piece of paper. Art may be one of the few outlets of self-expression available for this population.

Promotes Sublimation

There are too many idle hands and glazed minds, which are a direct result of the circumstances of having "nothing to do." Unacceptable behaviors triggered by emotions may be transformed into acceptable actions as these emotions are released onto a sheet of paper. In addition to their disease, Alzheimer's patients are limited by the health care system in Alzheimer facilities. There is not necessary programming to meet the daily requirements for interactive activities and stimulation. I have witnessed residents yell, push, and hit each other as they talk about how bored they are. I have heard them say, "There is nothing to do around here!" Having resources available, such as an interactive art experience, can, and will, transform these frustrations and dangerous, aggressive behaviors into tangible art forms. In one group, I observed a nearly blind woman, visibly agitated, become soothed, by manipulating portions of play dough and shaping them into pancakes.

Alleviates Boredom and Daytime Sleepiness

Having interactive art materials available to touch and manipulate focuses the patient's attention on pleasurable and self-soothing experiences. Each material evokes different responses and offers opportunity for stimulation, focus, and pleasure.

Promotes Connecting

Patients make contact with the materials as well as with other group members. Working in art gives patients a topic of conversation with one another as well as with the group leader.

Honors Capabilities and Integrity

Personality, character, and style become visible as patients begin to make their marks and create images. The power of these images may be a loud, strong voice of their inner experience.

Encourages Focus

Art tasks that are safe, engaging, and enjoyable are important ingredients to a successful art therapy program. Tasks need to meet the needs of the individual and must take into account his/her cognitive and physical capabilities. All art experiences must be designed to enable the patient to have a positive experience, independent of his/her limitations. Art experiences that utilize materials such as torn paper, photographs, paint, or clay, are the beginnings of a successful art therapy program. These experiences must capitalize on what the patient is able to do and the movements he/she can make.

The ability of the therapist, or other staff, to be flexible and shift from one frame of reference to another, as well as to be able to adapt to the specific needs and capabilities of the Alzheimer's patient, is imperative in response to the various stages in which the patients may be.

The artwork created in the group, if possible, should be displayed publicly at the facility, for family, friends, and staff to see. For some family members, visiting a loved one with Alzheimer's disease is difficult. They don't know what to say, what to do, or how to be with their loved one. This feeling, at times, keeps the family member from visiting. Making art together or viewing the creations of their loved ones helps diffuse this discomfort and awkwardness.

Conducting an Art Therapy Group with Alzheimer's Patients

As an Art Therapy Consultant in adult day care facilities, retirement communities, assisted living facilities, nursing homes, and Alzheimer's sheltered care units, I have had the privilege of creating meaningful art with older adults. I have seen bits of fabric transformed into a clothesline of memories, bits of paper symbolize a loved pet, or smiles of glee appear as blue watercolor paint reminds one of swimming. With the proper set up of interactive art materials, Alzheimer's patients have an avenue for self-expression. This invites individuals to break some of the repetitive cycles that increase with severity of the disease.

Additionally, it is important to understand that each group has a life of its own and needs to be thoughtfully designed to meet the individual client's needs. The groups may be high functioning, low functioning, or a mixture. The art therapist must guide individuals gently and supportively without undermining their self-confidence or intruding upon their personal territory.

Prototype of an Art Therapy Group Session

The following is a general description of a prototype of an art therapy group session with patients who vary in stages of Alzheimer's disease and related illnesses. It is, therefore, crucial to train nurses, aides, and volunteers to be supportive and aware of the art therapy program and its goals, so as to minimize the possibility that the staff will act in a way that diminishes, rather than enhances, possibilities for the residents. It takes a long time to establish this much-needed team approach. It is important to have therapist and staff work together towards enhancing experiential art therapy for the residents. Proper training of the staff can shift the staff atmosphere from apathy and burnout to stimulation and pleasure. In this way, the avenue of an art experience becomes a natural and regular part of the residents' day.

While working with a group, I constantly observe the hands of its members to evaluate their motor capabilities. I am thus able to attend to each individual's particular style and needs. We work together to build, construct, or draw their personal, emotional rhythm and reality. I focus on the process of making art as opposed to the result of the effort, thus on art as therapy rather than art psychotherapy. I perceive my role as an art therapist, in this setting, to be that of a creative coach. Many times I have to encourage reticent, resistant, fearful individuals to engage in the spontaneous art making of the group.

Set-up

It is vital for art therapists to be able to observe the total process. The role of the therapist is to assist clients to achieve some level of success in their projects/tasks. The length of an individual task may vary from five to 60 minutes or more.

The group room should be set up with tables and chairs with enough space to accommodate wheelchairs or other mobility aids. During my groups at each place there is a piece of white, 18"x 24" drawing paper, which can be taped to the table for stability. In the middle of the table is a collection of variously colored markers or oil pastels.

Warm-up Exercise

Some group members can't wait to get started. For others, facing the blank paper surrounded by drawing materials may be daunting. Familiar movements help patients to overcome this barrier. The first thing I do is have each participant select a colored marker or oil pastel and hold it in their dominant hand. Then I ask them to watch me and mimic my movements. I hold a marker or oil pastel in my hand and wave, wiggle, and stretch my arms gently in the air while telling them to move their hands like leaves blowing in the wind, like a rainstorm, or like a conductor. I encourage the patients to verbalize their perception of the movements while we are doing them. I do this for approximately two minutes. I then have them change the marker or oil pastel to the other hand and repeat the process. I then encourage them to make marks on the paper using the same hand motions they just used in the above exercise.

Utilizing line, shape, and color with swift strong strokes, group members begin to create images. They establish a pattern of movement and apply it to the page. I assist them in this as well as in switching colors and hands. The purpose of the warm-up exercise is to help individuals to transform inner motion onto a piece of paper.

Encouragement Exercise

After the warm-up, I circulate to each participant and continue to encourage them to expand on the marks they have just established. Different warm-up techniques may be experimented with. There are infinite ways to stimulate the older adult with Alzheimer's as well as the staff. The environment of the room should emanate aliveness and culture.

Discussion/Process

When we finish the images we go though a processing exercise. In this exercise, I hold up each image and coach a group discussion. Some of the questions that I ask are, "What does it feel like to be inside of this image? What is the line quality like? What do you see when you look at this? What kind of music would be playing? What does this remind you of? What title would you give this?"

This discussion is an important part of working with a person who has Alzheimer's. This part of a session validates the members and gives them a feeling of self-worth, and the sense that the marks and images they make have value. Group members usually respond positively to the other participant's art. This gives the artist positive reinforcement and validation. It is saying, "I see you and you have value" to a person who might have initially felt rather insignificant, worthless, or lost.

During the discussion period, with my coaching to respond to the artwork, words, sentences, and poetic statements emerge from the participants. Some members are initially hesitant; however, once this process begins, the comments range from playful to profound. I record many of these utterances during the group process. Often they can be organized and structured as poetry. Below are two examples of poems created in this way.

A Field of Dandelions

Swirls of color, big burst of yellow
Dandelions blowing in the wind
A beautiful tornado
A forest of dandelions
They come up through the cracks
They just grow anywhere!

A Large Bird

Smocking and snapping
Determined
A dinosaur
Get out of his way
Give him his freedom.

CONCLUSION

I have been intimately involved with geriatric facilities for 15 years, as my mother needed different levels of care. From this experience, I have found that the need for appropriate interactive programming is imperative, especially as we are living longer. This is a great opportunity for creative arts therapists with their unique style, expertise, and zest to establish programs in nursing home facilities.

The chasm between technological advances in our country and sophistication of appropriate programming for our geriatric facilities is wide. My wish is to close that gap and to create programs to enhance the well-being of our older adults and their families through interactive creative expression. To me, it feels human to care for our parents in a way that honors their integrity. Conversely, it feels inhuman to put them away like prisoners awaiting their death.

In many facilities, the music that is playing satisfies the "rhythm" of the staff, rather than the need of the residents. When I visit my mother, during this final stage of her disease, I have to ignore the infantilizing and insulting activities that are planned for the residents. It often seems that activities are planned because they are mandatory requirements, with little relevance to the population toward which they are aimed. Certain activities such as doing puzzles or playing trivia confuses and frustrates residents even more. These activities do not please the residents, nor are they helpful. I do not consider myself an expert in the field of gerontology, nor do I wish to propose that art making can "cure all ills." I do know that art can provide meaning and solace when one's world is reduced to a mere existence with one day blending into the next.

Art therapy enhances well-being. It is a way to offer experiences that stimulate and invite nourishment rather than boredom and aggression toward others. Meaningful activities are crucial to the daily life of patients. Art therapy is not merely an activity to entertain and take up time—it is a means to create an attitude which encourages and honors the integrity of our older adults.

In preparation for this chapter, I sorted through my mother's artwork. I became aware that her images reminded me of the essence and spirit, which she, in her advanced stage of Alzheimer's, still seems to possess—or is it my imagination or wish? I treasure the images I have, which my mom created over the ten years while she was able to paint. I treasure them because these images mark her struggle, her grit, her passion, her fears, her confusion, and her acceptance. I was fortunate to grow up with a loving mother who gave me comfort when I was sick, supported me when I felt upset, and seemed always to make the best of whatever situation in which she found herself. Even now, at the very last stage of her disease, there seems to be an acceptance and ease of being. Making art with my mother was a healing and restorative process for both of us. Watching others make art provided, and still provides, a sense of usefulness and community for me.

My experience with my mother challenged me to create expressive arts programming for geriatric facilities. I hope that by reading about my experiences, you, too, will be stimulated to continue and broaden this important work.

Author's Note: This chapter is dedicated to my sweet mother, who died shortly after this chapter was written. She gave me the gift of love —the love of animals, music, art, and caring for other humans in need. It was through her caring that I was able to care for her when she was unable. This chapter is written to encourage all caregivers to utilize the creative arts in order to honor the integrity of those who suffer from the devastating impact of Alzheimer's disease.

REFERENCES

Alzheimer's Disease and Related Dementias Fact Sheet (version ED226Z) [Online brochure, from www.alz.org]. (1999). Chicago, IL: Alzheimer's Association.

Galatzer-Levy, R. & Cohler, B. (1993). *The essential other: A developmental psychology of the self.* New York, NY: Basic Books, a Division of Harper Collins Publishers, Inc.

Hardin, P. (1992). What are you doing with the rest of your life? Choices in Midlife. San Rafael, CA: New World Library.

Hellen, C. (1992). *Alzheimer's Disease: Activity-focused care.* Stoneham, MA: Andover Medical Publishers, a Division of Butterworth-Heinemann.

Rugh, M. (2001). Art, nature and aging: A shamanic perspective. In M. Farrelly (Ed.), *Spirituality and art therapy: Living the connection* (pp. 167). London: Jessica Kingsley Publications.

Seiden, D. (2001). *Mind over matter.* Chicago, IL: Magnolia Street Publishers.

Chapter 11

HOSPICE IN THE HOME: A CASE STUDY IN ART THERAPY

Judith Wald

A hospice provides care for persons in the last phase of life. Hospice care focuses on pain management and quality of life for people who are terminally ill, as well as support for their families. "Hospice care emphasizes pain and symptom control, emotional and spiritual support, and practical assistance with the many issues that arise when one is seriously ill" (Hospice of Westchester).

While one usually thinks of a hospice as a physical institution, often connected with a hospital, some communities provide hospice care in the home. The hospice I worked for provided palliative care and comfort to patients who were diagnosed with a life expectancy of six months or less, with the philosophy that most people prefer to spend their last days at home, in familiar surroundings, with their loved ones.

Referrals to a hospice come from patients, families, physicians, clergy, nurses, and hospitals. The patient's physician is the attending physician, while the hospice team develops a plan of care. "The team includes professionals and volunteers who address the medical, emotional, and spiritual needs of the hospice patient and family" (Hospice of Westchester). In addition, the hospice I worked for has a Complementary Care Program, of "comfort-oriented medical care and alternative therapies . . . to provide the best quality of life possible" (The Complementary Care Program of Hospice of Westchester). These included therapeutic massage, reflexology, hypnotherapy, guided imagery, music therapy, yoga therapy, Reiki, art therapy, and biofeedback. Referrals to art therapy came from a social worker.

ART THERAPY IN THE HOME

Art therapy was introduced to the family and patients in the Complementary Care brochure as "a way for people to sort out their feelings and cope with overwhelming emotions. An art therapist is trained to help people through drawing, painting, or simply looking at pictures and talking about their concerns. These techniques can provide a way for dying persons to identify their current emotions, cope with anxiety, reminisce with family and friends, and provide life review and closure for some issues." In my work with hospice patients, I have used drawing, painting, clay, and viewing pictures as the tools of art therapy. As in any therapy work, the first step is to make the client feel at ease, to develop a trusting rapport. Casual, friendly conversation begins the session, and continues throughout.

Working in a patient's home, one meets the patient in a comfortable, natural setting. As my patients are usually referred to me due to their past art ability and interest, their art and craftwork is often displayed on the walls. This provides an easy opening to conversation, and brings the focus directly on the client, but in a nonconfrontational manner as the artwork is the object of discussion. Each painting or craftwork usually has an interesting story and background, and I quickly learn about the patient's children through the paintings of him or her or perhaps of a deceased husband who took the photos on a vacation that led to the paintings.

I bring a variety of art media, and if the patient is reluctant to begin drawing, I suggest that we draw a picture together. As my patients are frail, there may be a reluctance to "make art" again, due to real problems of poor eyesight, hand-grasp pain, or other physical ailments. In this case, discussing the patient's paintings and viewing large art pictures serve to promote discussion, reminiscence, and pride. One patient said, "I spent the whole visit bragging about myself;" as she was referred to me for her depression, as well as for her physical illness, art therapy definitely made her feel better. Dr. Edwin Cassem (2001) suggests asking the patient, "As you look back, is there anything you are especially proud of?" to help rehabilitate their self-esteem. Finding out "Who she was at the top of her game" reminds us that the patient is this same person, but with an awful diagnosis. Paying the patient this respect is restorative (Cassem, 2001).

There are also other people to contend with in the home setting: a daughter-in-law arrives with groceries, another hospice worker comes during the session, and the home health aide is always present. The latter often keeps the radio, music, or TV on during the session, but usually at a lowered volume. Of course this may interrupt the patient's concentration, but it is important to "go with the flow" and accept these interruptions, in order to gain the trust and support of the others involved in the patient's care and everyday life. Bell states that "being flexible in an appropriate way to the uniqueness of each home environment, and the lifestyles of those people living together under the same roof, is an essential part of being able to respond therapeutically to the circumstances and needs of patients being cared for at home" (as cited in Sezaki and Bloomgarden, 2000, p. 284).

CASE STUDY

Anne was an 89-year-old woman with a diagnosis of Congestive Heart Failure (CHF). The reason for referral to an art therapist was social isolation, with the goal to communicate feelings openly. She had previously enjoyed arts and crafts. Anne was seen for art therapy once a week for 11 one-hour sessions, over a period of three and a half months. She lived in her house, together with an aide.

When I first met Anne, she appeared frail. She presented in a pleasant, friendly manner. Anne proudly pointed out portraits on the wall she said she had drawn. She was reluctant to begin drawing, but agreed that we work together on a house. She had a charming manner of covering up her deficits by telling me what to draw, rather than drawing herself. When she did draw, her frailty and poor eyesight were evident in her shaky lines and difficulty seeing light colors. Boundary confusion appeared in her mixing up the inside/outside of the house. She engaged in cheerful conversation of how she enjoyed a simple country cabin, such as we drew, in Maine for vacations. She became more involved in drawing and conversation; she responded positively to the visit with improved affect.

The next week, Anne was alert and focused. She again pointed out past artwork she had done, including the embroidered seat of a chair, and excellent framed drawings of her son and daughter when they were children. She said her daughter had died as an adult and left children; she did not wish to elaborate. Anne worked together with me on a drawing of a vase of flowers. Her crayon pressure was weak. She was very engaged in the process, directing where to place flowers, completing the picture in a careful, balanced manner. No more reminiscence took place, as she concentrated on her drawing.

At the following session, Anne complained of a mild headache and lack of energy. We had planned last week that she would sketch me wearing a hat, and she enjoyed viewing the hats I brought. Instead, Anne suggested finding an object in her cabinet as an artistic inspiration. We chose a ceramic bird, and worked together drawing the bird on a branch with leaves. Anne was more directive than participatory, though she was able to focus well and provide excellent suggestions of how to improve the picture. Anne was relaxed and enjoyed conversing. However, of note was her talking about the "lake-water people" that live in the water in Moosehead Lake, asking if I had seen them. I asked her if they were imaginary or real, and she said they were real, small, and lived under a large ledge. Otherwise, her conversation was reality-based.

During session 4, Anne again complained of a mild, persistent headache. She was friendly and interactive, asking about my weekend. Anne mentioned concern for a neighborhood boy who she said told her that the other children wouldn't play with him, and how she wished she could help. We decided to draw my house together, with Anne asking relevant questions about the placement of chimney, windows, and doors. She helped correct the perspective, was well-focused, and attentive to details. Her additions were made with weak pressure, and at times her eyes didn't see boundaries well. She was insistent on completing together a satisfactory drawing, announcing when it was finished.

At the next session, Anne was awaiting my arrival, in good spirits and alert. For the first time she had a plan for artwork. She had saved a paper towel printed with a picture of grapes and leaves to reproduce. She said I should draw the grapes, and she the leaves. She was meticulous in planning the placement on the page, insistent on a careful, exact copy. She appeared to feel empowered in the role of planner and art teacher. Anne tried various strategies, finally deciding to trace the overall shape. Next week we planned to work further on this picture. She also was proud to show me a stitchery she had made years ago.

We talked of the Twin Towers tragic terrorist destruction of the day before. Anne said she used to work nearby, doing clerical and secretarial work, and knew the area well; she had dined in the Windows of the World Restaurant on the top floor of the Towers.

The next week, Anne appeared especially attractive with a new haircut; she joked about her new hairdo and nail polish. She was alert again, and joined in a conversation about last week's World Trade Center disaster with appropriate affect and comments. We worked together on the drawing of grapes and leaves that Anne initiated last week. She enjoyed directing me, in a teacher-like role, in what and how to draw to improve the picture. Once she had a marker in her hand, she carefully added relevant improvements, working with concentration to balance the picture.

The following week, Anne was alert and cheerful, actively participating in conversation and drawing. She spoke of growing up on a farm in Vermont, playing the piano, adding that now her left hand "won't work." She again spoke of "the little lake people that look strange, have no noses, live under a ledge in lakes," asking if I saw them when I went swimming; this was apparently a fixed delusion. Anne was able to focus well on coloring the grapes we had outlined previously. She was careful and meticulous, erasing parts to improve the picture, adding details to make it three-dimensional.

During the next session, Anne was very alert and cooperative, pleasant, with a good sense of humor. Her memory was excellent; she had put aside a decorative hat she made to show me, as she remembered we had talked of her sketching me wearing a hat. She was able to concentrate for longer periods of time on coloring in the grapes previously begun, with minimal assistance from me. We conversed as she drew, about hobbies, interests, and recipes. During her lifetime, Anne had sewed, knitted, painted, played piano, and read about religion. She proudly showed me watercolor cards she made with another visitor, and plans for other cards.

The following week, Anne conversed as she worked on her drawing of grapes. She said she wasn't feeling well, bothered by a sore throat, which lowered her energy level. At times she asked me to help with the drawing, which she completed during this session. She was proud of it, and talked of framing it and hanging it up it the kitchen. Anne spoke of her family, addressing that she would probably move to a nursing home. She said she was sad about it, but appeared to accept it.

While most of her conversation was reality-based (she talked of broth-ers in Chicago, a daughter that passed away), she again mentioned "the funny odd little people that live under a large rock ledge by the water."

The following session, Anne appeared listless, but demonstrated good memory in recalling that I was away on vacation the previous week. She used friendly humor in our conversations. I suggested we use watercolors, to perhaps paint a fall scene. Anne instead suggested that I bring over a large green plant to paint. She was very exact in planning out the placement of the plant on the page, measuring care-fully. She mixed a special shade of green, and insisted that I start paint-ing, as she lacked energy. Once again she assumed an empowering teacher role of directing and complimenting my efforts. After careful consideration, she drew lightly the outline of a vase for the plant. She chose to paint it yellow with purple shading, an excellent artistic choice.

The next week Anne was alert, cheerful, and conversational. She was amenable to try a different medium—clay. This medium was intro-duced to keep her more actively involved, and to help exercise her hands. She learned that the more she squeezed the clay, the softer and more malleable it became. She talked of making a basket, a baby car-riage with a doll baby, but settled on making a head with a hat. This was the same subject of the portraits she had done of her children that were hanging on the wall. She made the basic shapes for the head and hat and responded well to suggestions of how to manipulate the clay—squeezing, rolling, banging, flattening. Anne was left with clay to experiment with during my two-week vacation absence. Unfortunate-ly, when I returned from my vacation, I learned that Anne had been moved outside of the agency's area, so I no longer could see her.

TRANSFERENCE AND COUNTERTRANSFERENCE

Anne reacted to me in a mixed manner, with regards to transfer-ence. At first she was naturally cautious and apprehensive to find out what I was about and what I wanted from her, with my bag of art sup-plies. She protected herself by her reluctance to draw, gradually agree-ing to a two-person drawing. As she became more familiar with me, she took a more assertive, directive role, telling me what and how to draw; she seemed to participate more in correcting my drawing, first verbally and then with her crayon. Who was the art teacher/therapist, she or I? She seemed to need and relish this empowerment role, as most of the time her aide or a relative were telling her what to do and what not to do. This helped her feel that she "still really matters" (Cassem, 2001), a boost to her self-esteem and dignity. At times she called me "Missy," in a grandmotherly role; other times I was her comrade in art. When she took the initiative to bring the still-life paper towel picture to draw, she had truly become involved in the art therapy process herself, rather than in a power struggle. Sezaki and Bloomgarden summarized how Gibson "notes how the art therapist can assist a person to retrieve independence through art making, giving the elder person an opportunity to gain self-esteem" (2000, p. 283).

My countertransferential feelings began when I got a phone message asking me if I would like to work with hospice as an art therapist. I was flattered that someone had recommended me for this position that I was not seeking. But my other reaction was that hospice is for the dying, and though I had much experience working with the elderly, I had never specifically worked with an end-stage patient, and thought it would be too depressing for me. It brought up my sad feelings of losing my parents and other family members, friends, and clients. I returned the phone call to the social worker, planning to tell her that I wasn't available, but could recommend other art therapists. However, after speaking with the social worker, learning about their special Complementary Care Program and that it was all home visits, not an institutional or hospital hospice, I became interested and accepted. I recalled enjoying working privately with an elderly woman who had liked to paint in her home, and recalled how special it was to see the patient in her real home environment, to meet the family, and to realize how appreciative the family was. Sezaki and Bloomgarden note that "it is generally agreed that the home is the least restrictive activity of all sites where the elderly live, allowing for diversity of treatment and ideas" (2000, p. 283).

Specifically about my reaction to Anne, I was concerned to find her to be frail, but thrilled that she was nevertheless full of life and spunk, especially as she became more comfortable with me. It was difficult to see her health vacillate from week to week, but I observed that the art therapy distracted her from her physical frailty and that her mood was elevated by the end of the visit. I learned that it was important to call right before coming for a visit, not just earlier in the day, as one day I was sent away because she took to her bed feeling too ill to sit up; it had saddened me to see her this way. Another time, there was no answer at the door as the aide had just taken her to the hospital, fearing a T.I.A. (stroke). On a more positive note, I was also witness to improvements in her physical condition and mental alertness. And our sessions ended not because of her death, but because she was moved to live with another family member out of state. Unfortunately, there was no opportunity for closure, as I learned about this move upon return from a two-week vacation. The reality is that there is, in most cases, no time for closure, as I am informed by a phone call from the agency of the death of one of my patients. This often comes "unexpectedly," after a positive session with a patient, but of course reminds me what hospice is—end of life palliative care, and brings me to mourn the person in my own manner.

CONCLUSION

[The hospice model] is concerned with being empathetic and with creating a relationship with dying persons rather than with making decisions for them. It is based on the premise that we should work with the person as a complete human being rather than attending primarily to the physical malfunctions of the body or in any way segmenting the person into distinct physical, social, psychological, or spiritual categories. (Lair, 1996, p. 4)

In summary, art therapy is an excellent addition as part of a holistic approach to improve the patient's quality of life at the end stage of life. The art therapy session can be an enjoyable time when the patient is engaged in conversation and is concentrating on a productive endeavor. The artwork gives the patient a sense of pride and helps maintain his/her dignity as a productive adult, even in the last phase of life. The patient is encouraged to take the lead in use of materials, subject matter, and approach. If conflictual issues arise, they may be worked through in the session. Signs of dementia, confusion, and delusions are shared with the treatment team. Most important, in working with older adults in art therapy, is that the patient feels he/she still really matters, and is a person, despite his/her illness.

REFERENCES

Cassem, E. (2001, May). *Palliation of suffering at the end of life.* Grand Rounds Lecture at New York Presbyterian Hospital, White Plains, NY.

Hospice of Westchester. (n.d.) *The Complementary Care Program of Hospice of Westchester.* [Brochure]. White Plains, NY.

Hospice of Westchester. (n.d.) *Hospice of Westchester.* [Brochure]. White Plains, NY.

Lair, G. (1996). *Counseling the terminally ill: Sharing the journey.* Washington, DC: Taylor & Francis.

Sezaki, S. & Bloomgarden, J. (2000). Home-based art therapy for older adults. *Art Therapy: Journal of the American Art Therapy Association, 17*(4), 283-290.

RECOMMENDED READINGS

Andrews, K., Brocklehurst, J. C., Richards, B., & Laycock, P.J. (1980). The prognostic value of picture drawings by stroke patients. *Rheumatology and Rehabilitation, 19*, 180-188.

Arrington, D. B. (1985). Expressive therapy with elders and the disabled: Touching the heart of life. *Art Therapy: Journal of the American Art Therapy Association, 2*(3).

Barnett, C. (1989). The conundrum of Willem de Kooning. *Art & Antiques, 11*, 63-73, 128.

Begley, S., Springen, K., Katz, S., Hager, M., & Jones, E. (1986, September 29). Memory: Science achieves important new insights into the mother of the muses. *Newsweek*, 48-54.

Bergland, C. (1982). The life review process in geriatric art therapy: A pilot study. *The Arts in Psychotherapy, 9*, 121-130.

Bertman, S. (1991). *Facing death: Images, insights, and interventions.* Bristol, PA: Taylor & Francis.

Bertman, S., Ed. (1999). *Grief and the healing arts: Creativity as therapy.* Amityville, NY: Baywood Publishing Co.

Burnside, I. (1984). *Working with the elderly: Group process and techniques* (2nd Ed.). Monterey: Wadsworth Health Sciences.

Butler, R. N. (1963). The life review: An interpretation of reminiscence in the aged. *Psychiatry, 26*, 65-76.

Butler, R. (1967). The destiny of creativity in later life: Studies of creative people and the creative process. In R. Kahana & S. Levin (Eds.), *Psychodynamic studies on aging: Creativity. reminiscing and dying.* New York: International University Press.

Byock, I. (1997). *Dying well: The prospect for growth at the end of life.* New York: Riverhead Books.

Carmi, S., & Mashiah, T. (1996). Painting as language for a stroke patient. *Art Therapy: Journal of the American Art Therapy Association, 13*(4),265-269.

Cheyne-King. S. E. (1990). Effects of brain injury on visual perception and art production. *The Arts in Psychotherapy, 17*, 69-74.

Clair, A. A. (1996). *Therapeutic uses of music with older adults.* Baltimore: Health Professions Press.

Clinifoto, J. (1973). When the stroke patient draws a picture: A due to disability. *Geriatrics, 28*, 101-105.

Conger, D. K. (1979). Art therapy with elderly stroke survivors. *New York State Art Teachers Association Bulletin, 11*, 5-13.

Corbett, L. (1984). The developmental tasks of old age. *The Journal of Medical Aspects of Human Sexuality, 18*(10), 30-47.

Couch, J. B. (1994). Diagnostic Drawing Series: Research with older people diagnosed with Organic Mental Syndromes and Disorders. *Art Therapy: Journal of the American Art Therapy Association, 11*(2), 111-115.

Couch, J. B. (1995). A comparison of art therapy assessments used with older people. Unpublished manuscript.

Couch, J. B. (1997). Beyond the veil: Mandala drawings by dementia patients. *Art Therapy: Journal of the American Art Therapy Association, 14*(3), 187-193.

Crimmens, P. (2001). Review: Story-making and creative group work with older people. *Art therapy: Journal of the American Art Therapy Association, (2)*, 171-172.

Cronin, S. M., & Werblowsky, J. H. (1979). Early signs of organicitiy in artwork. *Art Psychotherapy, 6*, 103-108.

Crosson, C. (1976). Art therapy with geriatric patients: Problems of spontaneity. *American Journal of Art Therapy, 15*, 51-56.

Cummings, J., & Zarit, J. (1987). Probable Alzheimer's disease in an artist. *Journal of American Medical Association, 11*, 258.

Davisson, S. A., Rush, J. C., & Fitzner, D. H. (1982). Older adult art students: Descriptive data for community program planning. *Educational Gerontology, 8*, 129-141.

Demmer, A. C. (1979). Techniques of group art therapy for the elderly in a psychiatric hospital setting. *New York State Art Teachers Association Bulletin, 29*(3).

Dennis, W. (1966). Creative productivity between the ages of 20 and 80 years. *Journal of Gerontology, 21*.

Dewdney, I. (1973). An art therapy program for geriatric patients. *American Journal of Art Therapy, 12*, 249-254.

Dodd, F. (1975). Art therapy with a brain-injured man. *American Journal of Art Therapy, 14*, 83-89.

Dohr, J. H., & Forbes, L. A. (1966). Creativity, arts and profiles of aging: A reexamination. *Educational Gerontology, 12*, 123-138.

Doric-Henry, L. (1997). Pottery as therapy with elderly nursing home patients. *Art Therapy: Journal of the American Art Therapy Association, 14*(3), 163-171.

Drake, M. (1988, September). Art media with aging adults: Views from near the finish line. *Gerontology, 11*(3), 1-4.

Engle, P., & Muller, E. F. (1997). A reflection on art therapy and aging. *Art Therapy: Journal of the American Art Therapy Association, 14*(3), 206-209.

Erikson, E., Erikson, J., & Kivnick, H. (1986). *Vital involvement in old age.* New York: W. W. Norton.

Fenton, J. F. (2000). Unresolved issues of motherhood for elderly women with serious mental illness. *Art Therapy: Journal of the American Art Therapy Association. 17*(1), 24-30.

Fidler, G., & Velde B. (1999). *Activities: Reality and symbol.* Thorofare, NJ: SLACK Inc.

Field, J. (1976). Art therapy in a neurological hospital in London. *American Journal of Art Therapy, 15*, 99-103.

Finney, P. R. (1994). A review of two art assessment tools in an adult day treatment center. *Art Therapy: Journal of the American Art Therapy Association, 11*(2), 154-156.

Genevay, B. & Katz, R. (1990). *Countertransference and older clients.* Newbury Park, CA: Sage Publications.

Genser, L. (1985). Art as therapy with an aging artist. *American Journal of Art Therapy, 23*, 93-99.

Gonen, J., & Soroker, N. (2000). Art therapy in stroke rehabilitation: A model of short-term group treatment. *The Arts in Psychotherapy, 27*(1), 41-50.

Gotterer, S. M. (1989). Storytelling: A valuable supplement to poetry writing with the elderly. *The Arts in Psychotherapy, 16*, 127-131.

Greenberg, P. (1987). *Visual arts and older people: Developing quality programs.* Springfield, IL: Charles C Thomas.

Gregoire, P. A. (1998). Imitation response and mimesis in dementia. *Art Therapy: Journal of the American Art Therapy Association, 15*(4), 261-264.

Harrison, C. (1981). Therapeutic art programs around the world-XlII: Creative arts for older people in the community. *American Journal of Art Therapy, 19,* 99-101.

Henley, D. (1986). Approaching artistic sublimation in low functioning individuals. *Art Therapy: Journal of the American Art Therapy Association, 4*(2), 67-73.

Hughston, G. A., & Merriam, S. B. (1982). Reminiscence: A informal technique for improving cognitive functioning in the aged. *International Journal of Aging and Human Development, 15*(2), 139-149.

Hubalek, S. K. (1996). *I can't draw a straight line: Bringing art into the lives of older adults.* Baltimore: Health Professions Press.

Innes, A. & Hatfield, K. (Eds.). (2002). *Healing arts therapies and person-centered dementia care.* London: Jessica Kingsley Publications.

Jensen, S. M. (1997). Multiple pathways to self: A multisensory art experience. *Art Therapy: Journal of the American Art Therapy Association, 14*(3), 178-186.

Johnson, C., Lahey, P. P., & Shore, A. (1992). An exploration of creative arts therapeutic group work on an Alzheimer's unit. *The Arts in Psychotherapy, 19,* 269-277.

Jungels, G. (1979). Art and the older adult. *The New York State Art Teachers Association Bulletin, 29*(3), 2-11.

Jungels, G. (1982). *To be remembered: Art and the older adults in therapeutic settings.* Buffalo, NY: Potentials Development for Health and Aging Services.

Kahn-Denis, K. B. (1997). Art therapy with geriatric dementia clients. *Art Therapy: Journal of the American Art Therapy Association, 14*(3), 194-199.

Kaminsky, M. (1978). Pictures from the past: The use of reminiscence in casework with the elderly. *Journal of Gerontological Social Work, 1,* 19-32.

Kaminsky, M. (Ed.). (1984). *The uses of reminiscence: New ways of working with older adults.* New York: Haworth Press.

Karr, K. (1985). How to care for, comfort, and commune with your nursing home elder. *Activities, Adaptations, & Aging, 7*(1), 86.

Keler, M. J. (1990). *Activities with developmentally disabled elderly and older adults.* New York: Haworth Press.

Kerr, C. C. (1999). The psycho-social significance of creativity in the elderly. *Art Therapy: Journal of the American Art Therapy Association, 16*(1), 37-41.

Keyes, M. F. (1985). *Inward journey: Art as therapy.* LaSalle, IL: Open Court.

Knapp, N. M. (1992). Tabulated review of diagnostic use of art as a preliminary resource for research with Alzheimer's disease. *American Journal of Art Therapy, 31,* 46-62.

Knapp, N. M. (1994). Research with diagnostic drawings for normal and Alzheimer's subjects. *Art Therapy: Journal of the American Art Therapy Association, 11*(2), 131-138.

Koch, K. (1977). *I never told anybody: Teaching poetry writing in a nursing home.* New York: Vintage Books, Random House.

Landgarten, J. (1983, Fall). Art therapy for depressed elders. *Clinical Gerontologist, 2*(1), 45-54.

Leonard, A. (1993). Art therapy with a left-hemisphere post-stroke patient. ln E. Virshup (Ed.), *California Art Therapy Trends.* (pp. 129-139). Chicago: Magnolia Street Publishers.

Levine, S. (1997). *A year to live: How to live this year as if it were your last.* New York: Bell Tower.

Lewis, M. I., & Butler, R. N. (1974). Life-review therapy: Putting memories to work in individual and group psychotherapy. *Geriatrics, 29,* 165-173.

Link, A. (1997). *Group work with elders: 50 therapeutic exercises for reminiscence, validation, and remotivation.* Florida: Professional Resource Press.

Malchidoi, C. (1992). Art and loss. *Art Therapy: Journal of the American Art Therapy Association, 9*(3), 114-118.

McNiff, S. (1992). *Art as medicine: Creating a theory of imagination.* Boston: Shambala.

Moore, V., & Wyke, M. (1984). Drawing disability in patients with senile dementia. *Psychological Medicine, 14,* 97-105.

Neimeyer, R. (1998). *Lessons of loss: A guide to coping.* New York: McGraw Hill.

Orr, P. P. (1997). Treating the whole person: A combination of medical and psychiatric treatment for older adults. *Art Therapy: Journal of the American Art Therapy Association, 14*(3), 200-205.

Parson, C. L. (1986). Group reminiscence therapy and levels of depression in the elderly. *Nurse Practioner, 11*(3), 68, 70, 75-76.

Parsons, V. (1998). *Simple expressions: Creative and therapeutic arts for the elderly in long-term care facilities.* State College, Pennsylvania: Venture Publishing, Inc.

Peck, M. S. (1997). *Denial of the soul: Spiritual and medical perspectives on euthanasia and mortality.* New York: Harmony Books.

Perry, R.C. (2000). Drawing from within: Art therapy can speak for–and heal–your residents. *Contemporary Long Term Care, 23*(11), 22-25.

Pratt, M., & Wood, M. J. (Eds.). (1998). *Art therapy in palliative cafe: The creative response.* London: Routledge.

Priefer, B. A., & Gambert, S. R. (1984). Reminiscence and life review in the elderly. *Psychiatric Medicine 2*(1), 91-100.

Rando, T. (2000). *Clinical dimensions of anticipatory mourning.* Champaign, IL: Research Press.

Ridker, C., & Savage, P. (1996). *Railing against the rush of years: A personal journey through aging via art therapy.* Pittsburgh: Unfinished Monument Press.

Ringold, F., & Rugh, M. (1990). *Making your own mark: A drawing and writing guide for senior citizens.* Tulsa: Coman Associates.

Rogers, N. (1993). *The creative connection: Expressive arts as healing.* Palo Alto, CA: Science & Behavior Books, Inc.

Rosin, A., Matz, E., & Carmi, S. (1977). How painting can be used as a clinical tool. *Geriatrics, 32,* 41-46.

Rugh, M. M. (1985). Art therapy with the institutionalized older adult. *Activities, Adaption, and Aging, 6,* 105-120.

Rugh, M. M. (1991, Spring). Creativity and life review in the visual arts: The transformative experience of Florence Kleinsteiber. *Generations,* 27-31.

Sandel, S. & Johnson, D. (1987). *Waiting at the gate: Creativity and hope in the nursing home.* New York: Haworth Press.

Schimmel, B. F., & Kornreich, T. Z. (1993). The use of art and verbal process with recently widowed individuals. *American Journal of Art Therapy, 31,* 91-97.

Schwartz, M. (1996). *Letting go: Morrie's reflections on living while dying.* New York: Walker & Co.

Scott-Alexander, G. (1998). *The art of the moment.* Sand Lake, NY: Glass Lake Studio.

Sezaki, S. & Bloomgarden, J. (2000). Home-based art therapy for older adults. *Art Therapy: Journal of the American Art Therapy Association, 17*(4), 283-290.

Shore, A. (1989). Themes of loss in the pictorial language of a nursing home. *The Canadian Art Therapy Association Journal, 4*(1), 16-32.

Shore, A. (1997). Promoting wisdom: The role of art therapy in geriatric settings. *Art Therapy: Journal of the American Art Therapy Association, 14*(3), 172-177.

Silver, R. A. (1975). Clues to cognitive functioning in the drawings of stroke patients. *American Journal of Art Therapy, 15,* 3-8.

Silver, R. A. (1976). Using art to evaluate and develop cognitive skills. *American Journal of Art Therapy, 16,* 11-19.

Silver, R. A. (1978). *Developing cognitive and creative skills through art.* Baltimore: University Park Press.

Silver, R. A. (1993). Age and gender differences expressed through drawings: A study of attitudes toward self and others. *Art Therapy: Journal of the American Art Therapy Association, 10*(3), 159-168.

Silver, R. A. (1999). Differences among aging and young adults in attitudes and cognition. *Art Therapy: Journal of the American Art Therapy Association, 16*(3).

Simon, R. (1981). Bereavement art. *American Journal of Art Therapy, 20*(4), 135-143.

Simon, R. M. (1985). Graphic style and therapeutic change in geriatric patients. *American Journal of Art Therapy, 24,* 3-9.

Skinner, B. F. (1983). Creativity in old age: The key to productivity is to change the environment. *Psychology Today,* 3.

Spaniol, S. (1997). Guest Editorial-Art therapy with older adults: Challenging myths, building competencies. *Art Therapy: Journal of the American Art Therapy Association, 14*(3), 158-160.

Spaniol, S. (1992). Is there a "Late Style" of art? Line us in human figure drawing by elderly people. *Art Therapy: Journal of the American Art Therapy Association, 9*(2), 93-95.

Strosser, A. (1984). To be remembered: Art and the older adult in therapeutic settings. *Art Therapy: Journal of the American Art Therapy Association, 1*(3).

Verson, K. (1993). *Time dance: Looking backward, moving forward: The "art" of reminiscence.* Chicago, IL: Center for Applied Gerontology

Wadeson, H. (1987). Residential care for the elderly. In H. Wadeson (Ed.) *The Dynamics of Art Psychotherapy.* New York: John Wiley and Sons.

Wald, J. (1983). Alzheimer's disease and the role of art therapy in its treatment. *American Journal of Art Therapy, 22,* 57-64.

Wald, J. (1984). The graphic representation of regression in an Alzheimer's disease patient. *The Arts in Psychotherapy, 11*(3), 165-175.

Wald, J. (1986). Art therapy for patients with dementing illnesses. *Clinical Gerontologist, 4*(3), 29-40.

Wald, J. (1986). Fusion of symbols, confusion of boundaries: Percept contamination in the artwork of Alzheimer's disease patients. *American Journal of Art Therapy, 3,* 74-80.

Wald, J. (1993). Art therapy and brain dysfunction in a patient with a dementing illness. *Art Therapy: Journal of the American Art Therapy Association, 10*(2), 88-95.

Weber, B. L. (1981). Folk art as therapy with a group of old people. *American Journal of Art Therapy, 20,* 47-52.

Weber, J. A., Cooper, K., & Hesser, J. L. (1996). Children's drawings of the elderly: Young ideas abandon old age stereotypes. *Art Therapy: Journal of the American Art Therapy Association, 13*(2), 114-117.

Weisberg, N. & Wilder, R. (1985). *Creative arts with older adults: A sourcebook.* New York: Human Sciences Press.

Weishaar, K. (1999). The visual life review as a therapeutic art framework with the terminally ill. *The Arts in Psychotherapy, 26*(3), 173-184.

Weiss, W., Schafer, D. E., & Berghorn, F. J. (1989). Art for the institutionalized elderly. *Art Therapy: Journal of the American Art Therapy Association, 6*(1), 10-17.

Weiss, J. C. (1984). *Expressive therapy with elders and the disabled: Touching the heart of life.* New York: Haworth.

Wilkinson, N., Srikumar, S., Shaw, K., & Orrell, M. (1998). Drama and movement therapy in dementia: A pilot study. *The Arts in Psychotherapy, 25*(3), 195-201.

Williams, Y. B. (1999). *The art of dying: A Jungian view of patients' drawings.* Springfield, IL: Charles C Thomas.

Wikström, B. M., Ekvall, G., & Sanström, S. (1994). Simulating creativity through works of art: A controlled intervention study on creative ability in elderly women. *Journal of Creativity, 7,* 171-182.

Yaretzky, Y., Levinson, M., & Kimchi, O. L. (1996). Clay as a therapeutic tool in group processing with the elderly. *Art Therapy: Journal of the American Art Therapy Association. 3*(4), 75-81.

Zeiger, B. (1976). Life review in art therapy with the aged. *American Journal of Art Therapy, 15*(2), 47-50.

INDEX

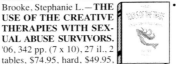

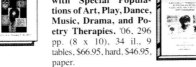
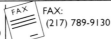

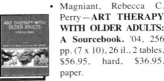

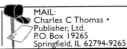
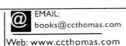